HYPERTHYROIDISM DIET COOKBOOK FOR BEGINNERS

Essential Nutritional Strategies to Balance Thyroid Function and Enhance Your Health

Kingsley Klopp

As a token of our gratitude for your purchasing our book, we will be providing you with extra bonuses.

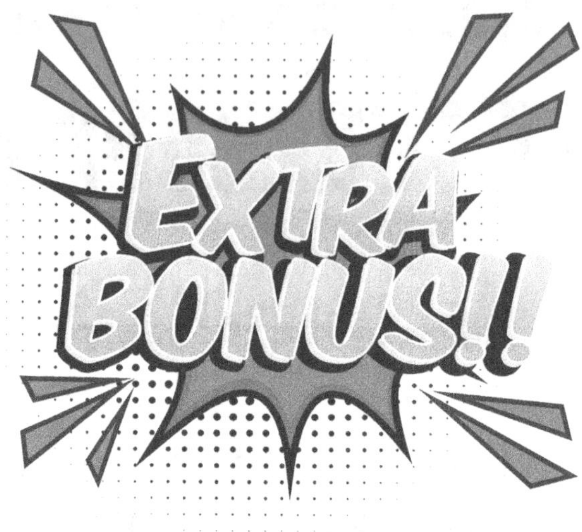

1. WEEKLY MEAL PLANNER JOURNAL
2. FREE E-BOOK FEATURING FULL-COLOR IMAGES OF THE FINISHED RECIPES.

Table of Contents

Fish Recipes

Desserts

SPECIAL NOTE

As you begin to explore these recipes, it's important to acknowledge that the journey of managing hyperthyroidism is highly personal. The way your body reacts to certain foods can be unique, and while our recipes aim to cater to common dietary needs associated with hyperthyroidism, your specific situation may require adjustments. We encourage you to use these recipes as a canvas, adapting them to your taste preferences and nutritional needs.

We recommend consulting with your healthcare provider to tailor these dishes perfectly for your health requirements, especially if you feel uncertain or if your symptoms persist. They can provide insights that align precisely with your medical history and current condition, ensuring that your diet is both safe and effective.

Please remember, the nutritional information provided with each recipe is an estimate based on standard ingredients and portions. Actual values can vary depending on the specific products used and modifications made. This flexibility allows you to explore substitutions and variations that not only satisfy your palate but also comply with your dietary needs.

Additionally, if this cookbook has enhanced your cooking and dining experience, we would love to read about your journey in an Amazon review. Conversely, if you encounter any issues with the recipes, please feel free to reach out to us at **kloppkingsley@gmail.com**. We are dedicated to assisting you throughout your culinary adventure.

Kingsley Klopp

Introduction

Welcome to a fresh start on your journey towards managing hyperthyroidism! If you've just been diagnosed, or have been living with this condition for a while, you know it presents unique challenges, especially when it comes to what you eat. But fear not, "Hyperthyroidism Diet Cookbook for Beginners" is your friendly companion, designed to demystify the foods and recipes that can support your health. This book isn't just a collection of recipes; it's a gentle hand guiding you through the often confusing landscape of nutritional needs when dealing with an overactive thyroid. Hyperthyroidism speeds up your metabolism, and managing it requires not just medication, but a thoughtful diet plan that complements your treatment. That's where we come in—offering you not just the "what" to eat, but the "how" and "why" behind each choice.

Each page of this cookbook is more than just a recipe—it's a conversation between friends. We understand that stepping into the kitchen can sometimes feel like navigating a minefield, especially when food sensitivities or symptoms like anxiety and increased heart rate step in. That's why we've put together not only mouthwatering recipes that cater to your condition but also tips on how to manage your symptoms through diet. Let's face it, changing your diet can be daunting. But think of this book as a friendly chat over coffee, where we explore new possibilities together. From understanding the role of iodine and selenium in your diet to figuring out which foods to avoid that might aggravate your thyroid, we cover it all in a simple and engaging way. Our recipes are designed to be simple, nourishing, and, above all, delicious. They cater to beginners, so you don't need to be a master chef to follow along. Whether it's a smoothie for a quick breakfast, a hearty soup for lunch, or a balanced dinner, our dishes are meant to bring satisfaction and health to your table. We also recognize that every person's experience with hyperthyroidism is unique. That's why we've included modifications for recipes wherever possible—to accommodate other dietary needs you might have, such as gluten-free or dairy-free options. It's all about making your journey as easy and enjoyable as possible.

Moreover, navigating your way through hyperthyroidism with this cookbook means you'll never have to go it alone. Consider this book a resource you can turn to again and again, whether you're looking for a quick snack or planning a special meal for friends and family who are eager to support your health journey. And beyond the recipes and tips, this cookbook encourages you to embrace a healthier lifestyle. With each dish, you're taking a step towards better managing your symptoms and improving your overall well-being. We'll explore together how balanced meals can help stabilize your energy levels and potentially ease some of the anxiety and sleep issues associated with hyperthyroidism.

So, put on your apron, and let's flip the page and begin this tasty and wholesome adventure together. With "**Hyperthyroidism Diet Cookbook for Beginners**" as your guide, you're well on your way to enhancing your diet and embracing a life full of energy and vitality. Welcome aboard— let's make your health the top priority it deserves to be!

Chapter 1: The Basics of Hyperthyroidism

WHAT IS HYPERTHYROIDISM?

Hyperthyroidism is more than just a medical term—it's a daily reality for many people. Imagine waking up each day feeling as if your body's internal engine is revving too high, too fast, with no off switch in sight. This is what life can feel like for someone with hyperthyroidism. At its core, hyperthyroidism occurs when your thyroid, a small, butterfly-shaped gland in the neck, becomes overactive. This gland has a big job: it regulates your metabolism, the process by which your body converts what you eat and drink into energy. In hyperthyroidism, the thyroid gland produces too much of its hormones, accelerating your body's metabolism unnaturally.

This acceleration can manifest in various ways. You might feel unusually anxious or irritable, almost as if you've had far too much caffeine. Your heart might race or flutter, even when you're sitting still. Sleep becomes elusive, and despite eating more than usual, you might find yourself losing weight without trying. For women, menstrual patterns can change, becoming lighter and less frequent. Others might notice a swelling at the base of their neck, a physical sign of the thyroid working overtime.
Living with hyperthyroidism often feels like being in a car where the gas pedal is stuck down, pushing you forward too quickly. It affects not just the physical body but also emotional and mental well-being. The constant rush can wear you down, making everyday tasks feel overwhelming. The journey to balancing thyroid levels often involves medication, dietary adjustments, and sometimes surgery or radioactive treatments, depending on the severity and cause. Each person's journey with hyperthyroidism is unique—what works for one might not work for another.

Despite the challenges, many with hyperthyroidism find paths to managing their condition and reclaiming their quality of life. Support from healthcare providers, loved ones, and community resources can provide a crucial network. Understanding and empathy from others can make a significant difference, turning a path fraught with challenges into a journey of healing and adaptation.

Understanding the Symptoms

Hyperthyroidism manifests through a variety of symptoms, each a reflection of the body's accelerated metabolic rate. Imagine your body like a machine that's always running at double speed—here are some of the signs that this might be happening:

- **Increased Heart Rate:** You might feel your heart pounding out of your chest, racing even when you're at rest. This isn't just a fleeting nervousness; it's a relentless feeling that can cause discomfort and anxiety.
- **Weight Loss:** Imagine eating more than usual, trying to sate a sudden, voracious appetite, yet your scale shows a decreasing number. This unexplained weight loss is a hallmark of hyperthyroidism, puzzling as it occurs despite increased food intake.
- **Heat Intolerance and Sweating:** You might find yourself intolerant to heat, the kind of person who is always turning down the thermostat or preferring to sit in the shade on a warm day. Excessive sweating accompanies this discomfort, even without exertion.
- **Tremors:** A fine tremor in your hands and fingers can be a subtle sign, like a barely noticeable shiver running through your palms, unsettling and seemingly unprovoked.
- **Mood Changes:** Hyperthyroidism can make you feel as if you're on an emotional rollercoaster—uncharacteristically irritable, anxious, or even depressed.
- **Fatigue and Muscle Weakness:** Despite high energy levels, there's an incongruous, profound fatigue, a kind of tiredness that rests deep in your bones, coupled with muscle weakness that makes everyday activities feel more strenuous.
- **Other Symptoms:** Women may notice changes in menstrual patterns, while others could experience increased bowel movements, or the appearance of a goiter—an enlargement in the neck caused by a swollen thyroid gland.

The Path to Diagnosis

Diagnosing hyperthyroidism involves a careful collection of puzzle pieces—symptoms, medical history, and diagnostic tests. Here's how the diagnostic journey typically unfolds:

- **Medical History and Physical Exam:** The process begins with a conversation. A healthcare provider will talk to you about your symptoms, medical history, and any family history of thyroid problems. They'll also conduct a physical exam, looking for signs like a swollen thyroid, tremors, and overactive reflexes.
- **Blood Tests:** The cornerstone of diagnosis is blood testing, specifically measuring levels of thyroid hormones—thyroxine (T4) and triiodothyronine (T3)—and thyroid-stimulating hormone (TSH). In hyperthyroidism, T4 and T3 levels are high, while TSH is usually low. This test not only confirms the condition but also helps gauge its severity.
- **Imaging Tests:** Sometimes, a picture is worth a thousand words. An ultrasound of the thyroid can help visualize changes in its structure, while a radioactive iodine uptake test can show how quickly the thyroid gland takes up iodine, a key component in hormone production. These images help in understanding the underlying cause of hyperthyroidism.
- **Additional Tests:** Depending on the initial test results and symptoms, additional tests might be required to explore further or to exclude other medical conditions that might mimic hyperthyroidism.

The Emotional and Practical Aspects

Being on the path to diagnosing hyperthyroidism can be emotionally taxing. The fluctuation in emotions, coupled with physical symptoms, can make patients feel as though they are not in control of their own bodies. Understanding these symptoms and the steps involved in diagnosis can empower you and demystify the process. This is not just about identifying a disease but about beginning a journey towards reclaiming your health and well-being.

Each step, from noting symptoms to undergoing tests, builds a clearer picture, aiming not just to label a condition but to pave the way for effective management and treatment. This journey, while sometimes daunting, is a critical path to improving quality of life and restoring balance in your body's intricate system of functions.

When someone is diagnosed with hyperthyroidism, the goal of treatment isn't just to slow the thyroid's overactivity but also to alleviate the profound impacts this condition can have on every facet of daily life. The approach to managing hyperthyroidism is often as multifaceted as the symptoms it presents, involving medication, possible surgery, and sometimes radioactive treatments, each tailored to individual needs and circumstances.

Medication

Medications are often the first line of defense in calming the hyperactive thyroid. Two primary types are commonly used:

- **Antithyroid Medications:** Drugs such as Methimazole or Propylthiouracil help slow the production of thyroid hormones. For many, starting these medications can feel like finally turning down a dial that's been stuck at maximum, reducing symptoms like anxiety, rapid heartbeat, and excessive sweating. These are typically used as a long-term treatment in many parts of the world, especially where radioactive iodine therapy is less favored.
- **Beta Blockers:** Although these drugs are generally used to manage high blood pressure, they are adept at controlling many of the uncomfortable symptoms associated with hyperthyroidism, such as tremors, palpitations, and anxiety. These don't stop thyroid hormone production but can make a significant difference in quality of life while other treatments work on the underlying condition.

Radioactive Iodine Treatment

Radioactive iodine therapy is another cornerstone of hyperthyroidism treatment. This approach uses radioactive iodine-131, taken as a pill, which directly targets thyroid cells. The treatment is straightforward: the iodine, because of its radioactive component, destroys overactive thyroid cells, thereby reducing hormone levels. For many patients, this treatment simplifies their condition into a more manageable form, often turning hyperthyroidism into hypothyroidism, which is easier to control with daily medication. The idea of using radioactivity can be daunting, but it has been used safely and effectively for decades.

Surgery

For some, when medication isn't suitable or if there's a significant goiter causing physical discomfort or cosmetic concerns, surgery might be the recommended route. The procedure, known as a thyroidectomy, involves removing part or all of the thyroid gland. Choosing surgery can be a significant decision, often bringing a mix of relief from symptoms and apprehension about undergoing a major medical procedure. Recovery from thyroid surgery typically involves hospital stay and careful monitoring, with the potential need for lifelong thyroid hormone replacement therapy.

Lifestyle Adjustments

Beyond medications and medical treatments, adjusting lifestyle can play a pivotal role in managing hyperthyroidism. Dietary changes can help support thyroid health and overall well-being. For instance, consuming foods rich in calcium and vitamin D is important, as hyperthyroidism can weaken bones. Reducing intake of iodine-rich foods, such as seaweed and other seafood, can also be beneficial.

Managing stress is another crucial element. High stress can exacerbate symptoms, making it essential to incorporate stress-reduction techniques such as yoga, meditation, or even simple daily walks, into your routine.

Support and Follow-Up

Living with hyperthyroidism often requires ongoing care and monitoring, involving regular check-ups with healthcare providers to ensure that treatments are effective and to adjust as necessary. This journey can sometimes feel lonely or overwhelming, so having a strong support network—whether through friends, family, or support groups—can make all the difference.

Each treatment plan is as unique as the individual experiencing hyperthyroidism. Doctors typically tailor treatments to best fit one's specific symptoms and lifestyle, aiming not just to treat the thyroid but to enhance a patient's overall quality of life. This patient-centered approach helps those with hyperthyroidism lead fuller, healthier lives, despite their diagnosis.

Chapter 2: Nutritional Foundations for Thyroid Health

ESSENTIAL NUTRIENTS AND MINERALS FOR THE THYROID

When it comes to the health of your thyroid—a small but mighty gland in the neck that governs metabolism—certain nutrients and minerals play a critical role. These substances are like the tiny, unseen workers helping to balance and optimize thyroid function, impacting everything from your energy levels to how your body uses food. Understanding which nutrients are essential and ensuring you get enough of them can be like fine-tuning an instrument, helping to produce the most harmonious symphony of bodily functions.

Iodine: The Keystone

Iodine is paramount for thyroid health. It's the core building block of thyroid hormones, thyroxine (T4) and triiodothyronine (T3), which regulate metabolism. The body doesn't produce iodine, so it must come from your diet. However, it's a delicate balance; both too little and too much iodine can lead to thyroid dysfunction. Including iodine-rich foods like seaweed, fish, dairy, and iodized salt in moderation can help maintain this balance.

Selenium: The Protector

Selenium is crucial for the conversion of T4 into the more active T3. It also protects the thyroid gland from oxidative damage due to its antioxidant properties. This mineral can be thought of as the bodyguard of the thyroid, warding off harmful invaders that can disrupt its function. Foods rich in selenium include Brazil nuts, tuna, sardines, eggs, and legumes. Integrating these into your diet can support your thyroid and overall antioxidant defenses.

Zinc: The Converter

Zinc aids in the conversion of T4 to T3 and is essential for the synthesis of thyroid hormones. Low levels of zinc can lead to reduced thyroid function. Zinc also supports the immune system, which is vital because thyroid health is closely linked to immune function. Foods high in zinc such as oysters, beef, chicken, tofu, and lentils can be valuable additions to your meals.

Iron: The Energizer

Iron deficiency can disrupt thyroid hormone synthesis by reducing the activity of heme-dependent thyroid peroxidase, the enzyme needed for thyroid hormone production. For those with hypothyroidism, iron is particularly important. Good sources of iron include red meat, poultry, lentils, and fortified cereals. Ensuring adequate iron intake can help maintain energy levels and support thyroid health.

Vitamin D: The Immune Modulator

Vitamin D's role in thyroid function is increasingly recognized due to its effects on the immune system and potential link to autoimmune thyroid diseases, such as Hashimoto's thyroiditis. Maintaining adequate levels of vitamin D through exposure to sunlight, foods like fatty fish and fortified milk, or supplements is crucial for thyroid wellness and overall immune resilience.

Magnesium: The Metabolism Manager

Magnesium is involved in numerous processes that regulate thyroid function. It helps manage T4 production and can calm the body, reducing stress, which is often high in thyroid dysfunction cases. Magnesium-rich foods include almonds, spinach, and avocados, which can help keep your metabolism running smoothly.

Incorporating These Nutrients

Adopting a diet that supports thyroid health doesn't just mean focusing on individual nutrients; it involves a holistic approach. Eating a balanced diet rich in fruits, vegetables, lean proteins, and whole grains can provide a broad spectrum of the nutrients your thyroid needs to function optimally. It's also about the emotional and social aspects of eating. Meals are not just for nourishment but are a source of joy and a means of connecting with others. By choosing foods that support thyroid health, you are not just feeding your body, but also nurturing your well-being and maintaining your social bonds.

Maintaining thyroid health through diet is an ongoing process, a continuous tuning of your daily nutrition to meet the unique needs of your body. It's a journey of discovery, learning which foods your body thrives on and which ones to avoid to feel your best. This journey, enriched by a variety of nutrient-dense foods, not only fuels your thyroid but also enhances your entire life, empowering you to live vibrantly and healthily.

Foods to Include
Focusing on foods that support overall health and potentially help regulate an overactive thyroid can create a foundation of nutritional balance:

- **Cruciferous Vegetables:** Broccoli, cauliflower, and kale may help manage thyroid function by impacting how the thyroid uses iodine. They can be particularly beneficial when eaten in moderation and cooked, as cooking helps reduce their goitrogenic properties (substances that can interfere with thyroid hormone production).
- **High-Fiber Foods:** A hyperactive thyroid speeds everything up, including the digestive system. This can lead to symptoms like frequent bowel movements. Foods rich in fiber such as berries, beans, and whole grains can help regulate digestion and improve gut health.
- **Proteins:** Lean proteins like chicken, turkey, and fish provide essential amino acids without excessive calories. They are vital for maintaining muscle mass, which can be lost due to an increased metabolism in hyperthyroid patients.
- **Dairy and Calcium-Rich Foods:** Since hyperthyroidism can accelerate bone turnover and lead to bone thinning, it's important to include calcium-rich foods in your diet. Dairy products, fortified plant milks, and leafy greens can help support bone health.
- **Healthy Fats:** Fats are crucial for overall health and can help manage the increased metabolism rate. Foods such as avocados, olive oil, and nuts provide essential fatty acids and calories needed for maintaining a healthy weight.

Foods to Avoid
Just as some foods can be beneficial, others might exacerbate hyperthyroid symptoms or the condition itself:

- **Excess Iodine:** While iodine is critical for thyroid function, too much can worsen hyperthyroidism. Avoiding iodine supplements and limiting high-iodine foods like seaweed and various seafoods can help keep your iodine levels in check.
- **Gluten:** If you have an autoimmune thyroid disorder like Graves' disease, which is a common cause of hyperthyroidism, gluten might exacerbate the problem. Many people find relief from autoimmune symptoms when they eliminate gluten from their diet.

- **Caffeine and Stimulants**: Caffeinated beverages and stimulants such as coffee, tea, and certain sodas can increase heart rate and exacerbate symptoms like nervousness and irritability. Opting for herbal teas or decaffeinated options can be more soothing.
- **Refined Sugars**: High sugar intake can lead to spikes in energy followed by crashes, which can be particularly hard on the thyroid and overall hormonal balance. Limiting foods high in refined sugars and opting for whole fruits and natural sweeteners may help maintain stable energy levels.

UNDERSTANDING FOOD LABELS AND THYROID TRIGGERS

When managing a condition like hyperthyroidism, understanding the language of food labels becomes more than just a skill—it's an essential part of navigating your health journey. For many, the supermarket is not just a place to shop; it's a terrain dotted with potential thyroid triggers, each packaged item holding clues about its impact on your condition. Developing the ability to decode these labels can empower you, turning the anxiety of food choices into a confident quest for well-being.

The Importance of Reading Labels

For those with hyperthyroidism, certain ingredients can exacerbate symptoms or interfere with medication efficacy. Learning to read food labels helps you avoid these compounds, making it easier to maintain balanced thyroid function. The process can seem daunting at first, with a list of ingredients more like a chemical inventory than a pantry list. But over time, label reading becomes a quicker, almost automatic task that enhances your ability to make informed choices.

Key Ingredients to Watch

- **Iodine:** This mineral is critical for thyroid function but can be a double-edged sword for those with hyperthyroidism. Too much iodine can aggravate the thyroid, leading to increased hormone production. Food labels might not always list iodine content directly, unless it's added as a supplement, but be wary of foods known to be high in iodine, such as dairy products, seafood, and iodized salt.
- **Soy:** While soy is often praised for its health benefits, it contains isoflavones that may act as goitrogens—substances that can interfere with thyroid hormone production. This doesn't mean you need to avoid soy entirely, but if you have hyperthyroidism, it's wise to consume it in moderation and not as a primary protein source.
- **Gluten:** For those with autoimmune thyroid disorders like Graves' disease, gluten can sometimes trigger an immune response that may worsen thyroid dysfunction. Checking labels for gluten—a common ingredient in many processed foods—is crucial. It's found not only in obvious products like bread and pasta but also in many sauces, condiments, and snack foods.
- **Artificial Additives:** Certain additives and preservatives may increase hyperthyroid symptoms or impact overall health. For example, aspartame, an artificial sweetener, has been reported to cause anxiety and irritability in some people, compounding similar symptoms often experienced in hyperthyroidism.

The Art of Label Reading
Reading a food label effectively requires more than just scanning for a few keywords. It involves understanding the nutritional content—identifying high-fiber options, recognizing high-quality protein sources, and spotting low-iodine choices. Here's how you can make the most of this information:

1. **Start with the Serving Size:** All the nutritional information on the label is based on the serving size, often much smaller than what people typically consume in one sitting.
2. **Check the Ingredients List:** Ingredients are listed in order of quantity, from highest to lowest. Look for whole foods as the first ingredients and be mindful of hidden sources of iodine, gluten, and soy.
3. **Identify Nutrient Content:** Pay attention to sodium (which might indicate processed foods high in additives), sugars, and types of fat. Opting for foods with unsaturated fats, low sugar, and minimal added sodium can contribute to better overall health and thyroid function.
4. **Look for Certifications:** Labels like "gluten-free," "organic," or "non-GMO" can help guide choices, especially for those with specific dietary needs related to their thyroid condition.

Personalization and Support
Adapting to a diet that considers thyroid health can feel isolating at times, but it also opens up a community of others navigating similar paths. Online forums, support groups, and nutritionists specializing in thyroid health can offer advice and camaraderie as you learn to translate the language of food labels into your everyday choices.

Reading food labels is not just a technical skill—it's a practice in mindfulness, empowering you to make choices that nurture rather than challenge your health. With each grocery trip, you become more adept at avoiding thyroid triggers and more engaged with your dietary needs, transforming your diet into one of the most potent tools you have to manage your hyperthyroidism. This proactive approach not only supports your physical health but also reinforces a sense of control and well-being in your journey with hyperthyroidism.

Breakfast Recipes

1. Herbed Mushroom and Kale Frittata

Ingredients:

- 8 large eggs
- 1/2 cup milk (use almond or coconut milk for a dairy-free option)
- 1 cup chopped kale, stems removed
- 1 cup sliced mushrooms
- 1/2 onion, diced
- 2 cloves garlic, minced
- 1 tbsp olive oil
- 1/2 tsp salt
- 1/4 tsp black pepper
- 1 tbsp fresh thyme, chopped
- 1 tbsp fresh parsley, chopped

Instructions:

1. Preheat the oven to 375°F (190°C).
2. In a medium skillet, heat olive oil over medium heat. Add the onion and garlic, and sauté until the onion is translucent.
3. Add the mushrooms and cook until they are golden brown.
4. Stir in the kale and cook until it is wilted.
5. In a large bowl, whisk together the eggs, milk, salt, pepper, thyme, and parsley.
6. Add the cooked vegetables to the egg mixture and stir to combine.
7. Pour the mixture into a greased 9-inch pie dish.
8. Bake in the preheated oven for 25-30 minutes, or until the eggs are set and the top is lightly golden.
9. Let cool for a few minutes before slicing.

Nutrition Info Per Serving (Serves 6):

- Calories: 140
- Fat: 10g
- Carbohydrates: 4g
- Protein: 9g
- Sodium: 300mg

Cooking Time:

- Preparation time: 15 minutes
- Cooking time: 30 minutes
- Total time: 45 minutes

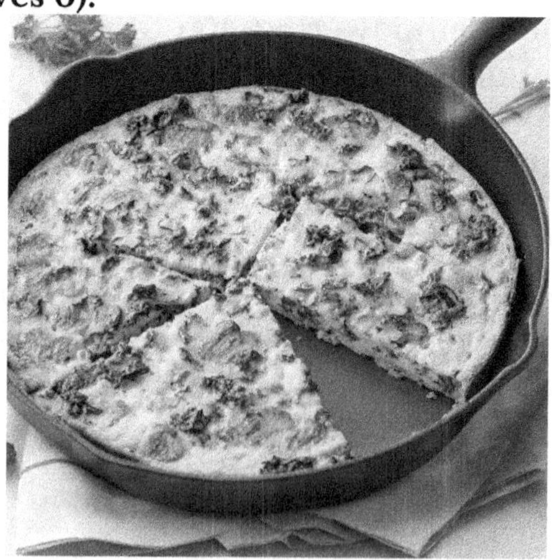

2. Coconut Yogurt Parfait with Mango and Pineapple

Ingredients:

- 1 cup coconut yogurt
- 1/2 cup diced mango
- 1/2 cup diced pineapple
- 1/4 cup granola (gluten-free if necessary)
- 1 tbsp honey or maple syrup (optional)
- Mint leaves for garnish (optional)

Instructions:

1. In a serving glass or bowl, layer half of the coconut yogurt at the bottom.
2. Add a layer of half the mango and half the pineapple.
3. Sprinkle half of the granola over the fruit.
4. Drizzle with a little honey or maple syrup if using.
5. Repeat the layers with the remaining ingredients.
6. Garnish with mint leaves if desired.
7. Serve immediately or chill in the refrigerator until ready to eat.

Nutrition Info Per Serving (Serves 2):

- Calories: 200
- Fat: 8g
- Carbohydrates: 30g
- Protein: 5g
- Sodium: 60mg

Cooking Time:

- Preparation time: 10 minutes
- Total time: 10 minutes

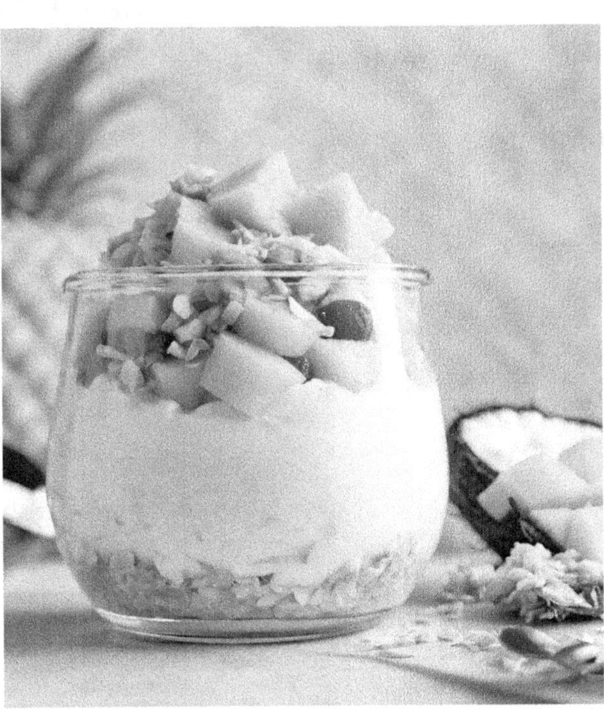

3. Warm Barley Cereal with Honey and Spices

Ingredients:

- 1 cup hulled barley, rinsed
- 4 cups water
- 1/2 tsp salt
- 1/2 tsp cinnamon
- 1/4 tsp nutmeg
- 1/4 tsp cardamom
- 2 tbsp honey
- 1/2 cup milk (almond or coconut milk for a dairy-free option)
- Fresh berries or chopped nuts for topping (optional)

Instructions:

1. In a medium saucepan, combine barley, water, and salt. Bring to a boil over high heat.
2. Reduce heat to low and simmer, covered, for about 30 minutes or until barley is tender and most of the water is absorbed.
3. Stir in cinnamon, nutmeg, cardamom, and honey. Mix well.
4. Add milk and continue to cook for another 5 minutes, stirring occasionally.
5. Serve hot, topped with fresh berries or chopped nuts if desired.

Nutrition Info Per Serving (Serves 4):

- Calories: 180
- Fat: 2g
- Carbohydrates: 40g
- Protein: 4g
- Sodium: 300mg

Cooking Time:

- Preparation time: 5 minutes
- Cooking time: 35 minutes
- Total time: 40 minutes

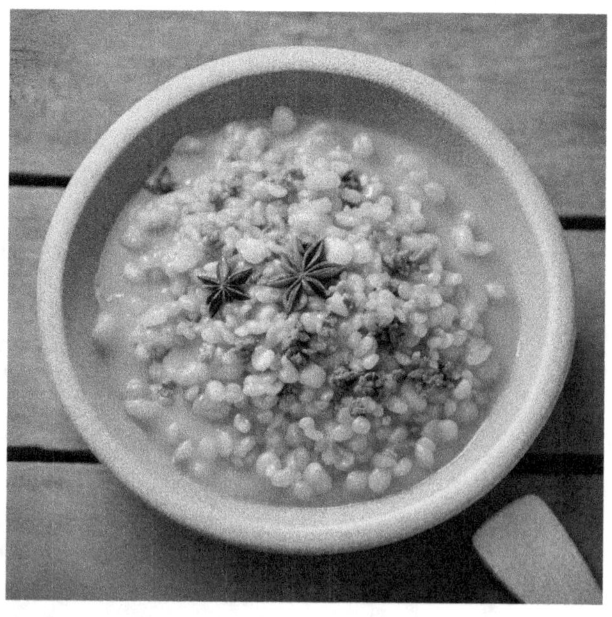

4. Multi-grain Porridge with Maple Syrup and Almonds

Ingredients:

- 1/4 cup rolled oats
- 1/4 cup quinoa
- 1/4 cup millet
- 4 cups water or milk (almond or soy milk for a vegan option)
- 1/4 tsp salt
- 2 tbsp maple syrup
- 1/4 cup sliced almonds
- Fresh fruits for topping (optional)

Instructions:

1. Combine oats, quinoa, millet, and salt with water or milk in a large saucepan. Bring to a boil.
2. Reduce heat to low and simmer, stirring occasionally, for about 20 minutes or until the grains are tender and creamy.
3. Remove from heat and stir in maple syrup.
4. Serve in bowls, topped with sliced almonds and fresh fruits if desired.

Nutrition Info Per Serving (Serves 4):

- Calories: 220
- Fat: 5g
- Carbohydrates: 38g
- Protein: 8g
- Sodium: 150mg

Cooking Time:

- Preparation time: 5 minutes
- Cooking time: 20 minutes
- Total time: 25 minutes

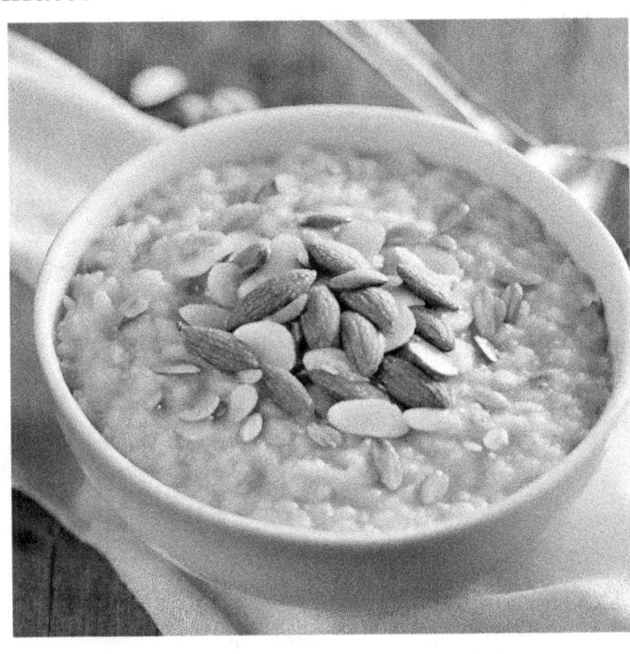

5. Pumpkin Oatmeal Cookies

Ingredients:

- 1 cup rolled oats
- 1/2 cup whole wheat flour
- 1/4 tsp baking soda
- 1/4 tsp salt
- 1 tsp cinnamon
- 1/2 tsp nutmeg
- 1/4 cup unsalted butter, softened
- 1/4 cup brown sugar
- 1/4 cup pumpkin puree
- 1 egg
- 1 tsp vanilla extract
- 1/2 cup raisins (optional)

Instructions:

1. Preheat the oven to 350°F (175°C).
2. In a small bowl, mix together the oats, flour, baking soda, salt, cinnamon, and nutmeg.
3. In a larger bowl, beat together the butter, brown sugar, pumpkin puree, egg, and vanilla until smooth.
4. Gradually add the dry ingredients to the wet, mixing until just combined. Fold in raisins if using.
5. Drop tablespoonfuls of the dough onto a baking sheet lined with parchment paper.
6. Bake for 12-15 minutes, or until the edges are golden.
7. Allow to cool on the baking sheet for 5 minutes before transferring to a wire rack to cool completely.

Nutrition Info Per Serving (Makes 12 cookies):

- Calories: 100
- Fat: 4g
- Carbohydrates: 15g
- Protein: 2g
- Sodium: 75mg

Cooking Time:

- Preparation time: 10 minutes
- Cooking time: 15 minutes
- Total time: 25 minutes

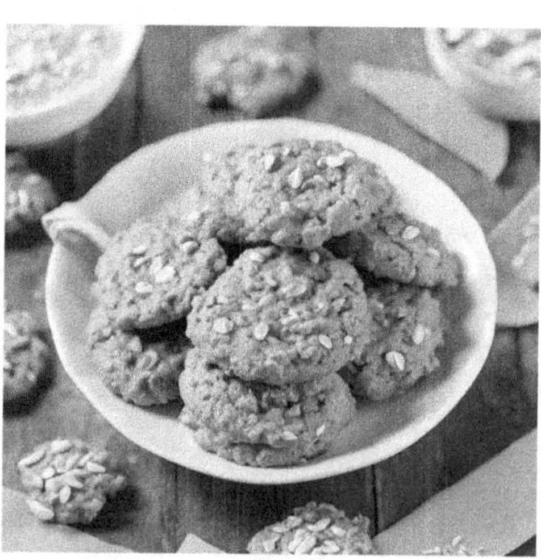

6. Sprouted Bean and Avocado Salad

Ingredients:

- 2 cups sprouted beans (such as lentils, chickpeas, or mung beans)
- 1 ripe avocado, diced
- 1 small red onion, finely chopped
- 1 tomato, diced
- 1 cucumber, diced
- Juice of 1 lime
- 2 tbsp olive oil
- Salt and pepper to taste
- Fresh cilantro, chopped (optional)

Instructions:

1. In a large bowl, combine the sprouted beans, avocado, red onion, tomato, and cucumber.
2. In a small bowl, whisk together lime juice, olive oil, salt, and pepper.
3. Pour the dressing over the salad and toss gently to coat.
4. Garnish with fresh cilantro if desired.
5. Serve immediately or chill in the refrigerator before serving.

Nutrition Info Per Serving (Serves 4):

- Calories: 250
- Fat: 15g
- Carbohydrates: 23g
- Protein: 8g
- Sodium: 150mg

Cooking Time:

- Preparation time: 15 minutes
- Total time: 15 minutes

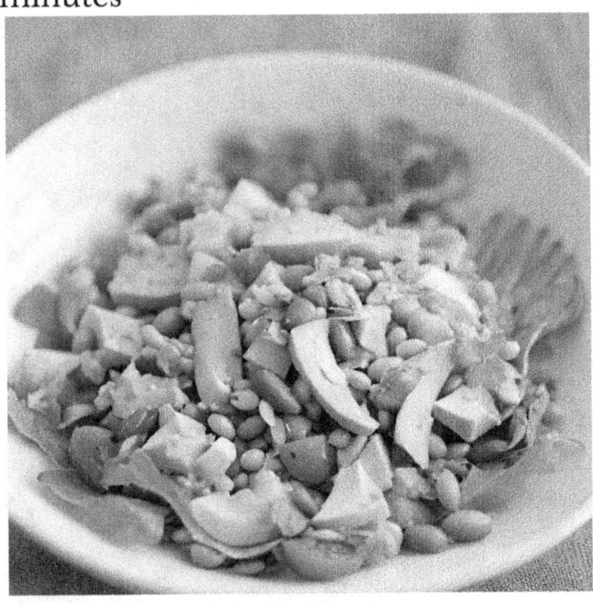

7. Bulgur Wheat Pilaf with Dried Apricots and Nuts

Ingredients:

- 1 cup bulgur wheat
- 2 cups water
- 1/2 tsp salt
- 1/2 cup dried apricots, chopped
- 1/4 cup chopped almonds
- 1/4 cup chopped walnuts
- 1/4 cup chopped fresh parsley
- 2 tbsp olive oil
- Juice of 1 lemon

Instructions:

1. In a saucepan, bring water and salt to a boil. Add bulgur wheat, cover, and reduce heat to low.
2. Simmer for 12-15 minutes or until all water is absorbed.
3. Fluff the bulgur with a fork and stir in olive oil, lemon juice, apricots, almonds, walnuts, and parsley.
4. Serve warm or at room temperature.

Nutrition Info Per Serving (Serves 4):

- Calories: 290
- Fat: 14g
- Carbohydrates: 38g
- Protein: 7g
- Sodium: 300mg

Cooking Time:

- Preparation time: 5 minutes
- Cooking time: 15 minutes
- Total time: 20 minutes

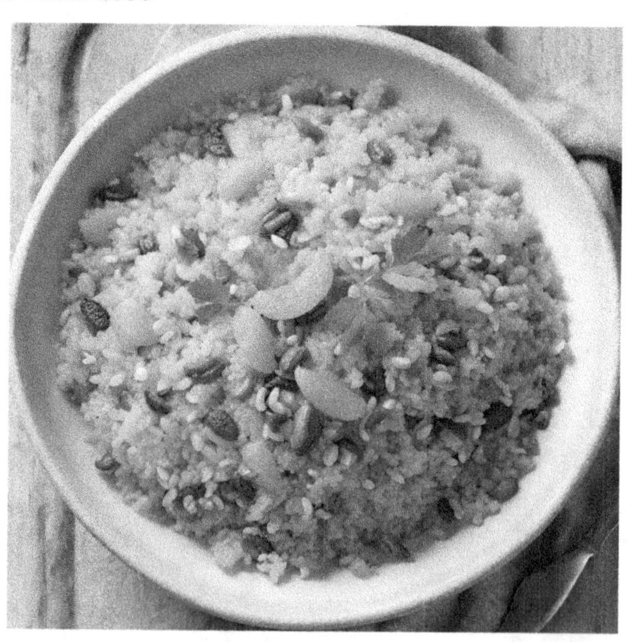

8. Whole Wheat Vegetable Pita Pocket

Ingredients:

- 4 whole wheat pita breads
- 1 cup hummus
- 1 bell pepper, sliced
- 1 small cucumber, sliced
- 1 tomato, sliced
- 1 small red onion, sliced
- 1 cup mixed greens (lettuce, spinach, or arugula)
- Salt and pepper to taste

Instructions:

1. Warm the pita breads in a toaster or oven until slightly crisp.
2. Cut each pita in half and spread hummus inside each half.
3. Stuff each pita half with bell pepper, cucumber, tomato, onion, and mixed greens.
4. Season with salt and pepper to taste.
5. Serve immediately.

Nutrition Info Per Serving (Serves 4):

- Calories: 300
- Fat: 9g
- Carbohydrates: 47g
- Protein: 12g
- Sodium: 600mg

Cooking Time:

- Preparation time: 10 minutes
- Total time: 10 minutes

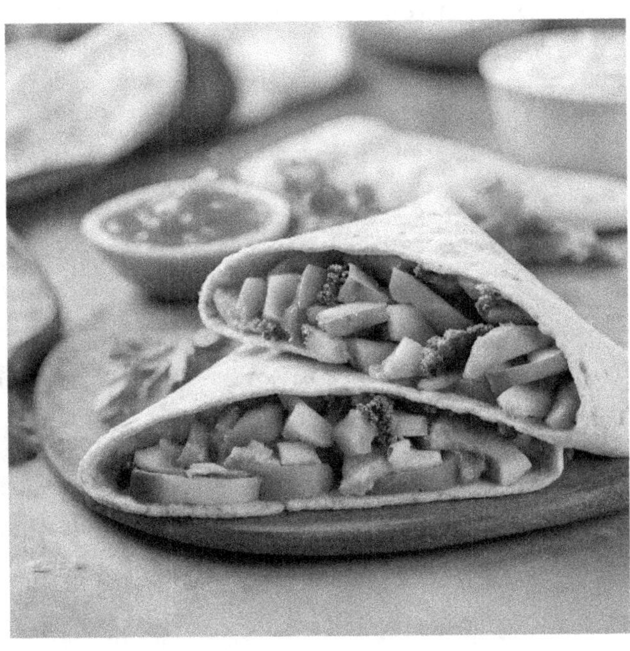

9. Tofu Scramble with Spinach and Sweet Peppers

Ingredients:

- 1 block (14 oz) firm tofu, drained and crumbled
- 2 cups fresh spinach, chopped
- 1 red sweet pepper, diced
- 1 yellow sweet pepper, diced
- 1 onion, diced
- 2 cloves garlic, minced
- 1 tsp turmeric
- 1/2 tsp black pepper
- 1 tbsp olive oil
- Salt to taste

Instructions:

1. Heat olive oil in a skillet over medium heat.
2. Add onion and garlic, sauté until onions are translucent.
3. Add sweet peppers and cook for another 5 minutes until softened.
4. Stir in crumbled tofu, turmeric, black pepper, and salt. Cook for 5-7 minutes, stirring frequently.
5. Add chopped spinach and cook until wilted, about 2 minutes.
6. Serve hot.

Nutrition Info Per Serving (Serves 4):

- Calories: 150
- Fat: 9g
- Carbohydrates: 10g
- Protein: 12g
- Sodium: 200mg

Cooking Time:

- Preparation time: 10 minutes
- Cooking time: 15 minutes
- Total time: 25 minutes

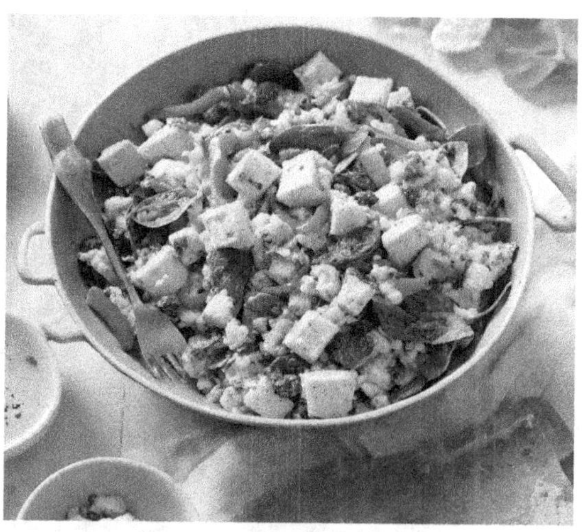

10. Savory Millet and Vegetable Bowl

Ingredients:

- 1 cup millet
- 2 cups vegetable broth
- 1 zucchini, chopped
- 1 carrot, chopped
- 1 bell pepper, chopped
- 1/2 cup frozen peas
- 1 tbsp olive oil
- Salt and pepper to taste
- Fresh herbs (such as parsley or cilantro), chopped

Instructions:

1. Rinse millet under cold water. In a saucepan, bring vegetable broth to a boil. Add millet, reduce heat to low, cover, and simmer for 20 minutes.
2. In a separate skillet, heat olive oil over medium heat. Add zucchini, carrot, and bell pepper; sauté until tender.
3. Stir in peas and cook until heated through.
4. Combine cooked vegetables with millet, season with salt and pepper, and mix well.
5. Garnish with fresh herbs before serving.

Nutrition Info Per Serving (Serves 4):

- Calories: 260
- Fat: 5g
- Carbohydrates: 47g
- Protein: 7g
- Sodium: 300mg

Cooking Time:

- Preparation time: 10 minutes
- Cooking time: 30 minutes
- Total time: 40 minutes

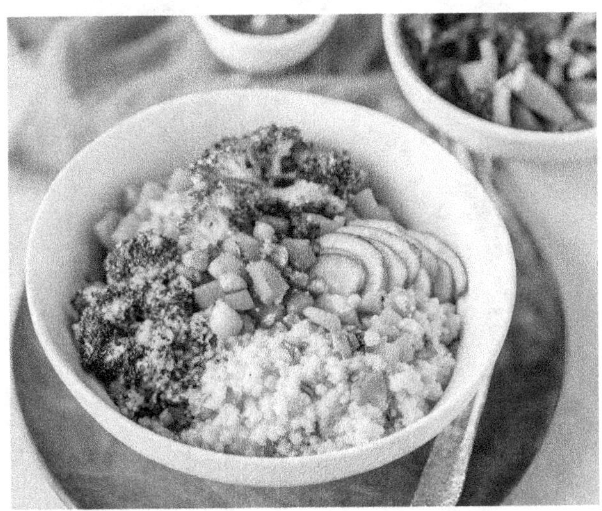

11. Mixed Berry and Flaxseed Smoothie

Ingredients:

- 1 cup frozen mixed berries (blueberries, raspberries, strawberries)
- 1 banana
- 1 tbsp ground flaxseed
- 1 cup almond milk
- 1 tbsp honey (optional)

Instructions:

1. Place all ingredients in a blender.
2. Blend on high until smooth.
3. Serve immediately.

Nutrition Info Per Serving (Serves 2):

- Calories: 180
- Fat: 3g
- Carbohydrates: 35g
- Protein: 3g
- Sodium: 90mg

Cooking Time:

- Preparation time: 5 minutes
- Total time: 5 minutes

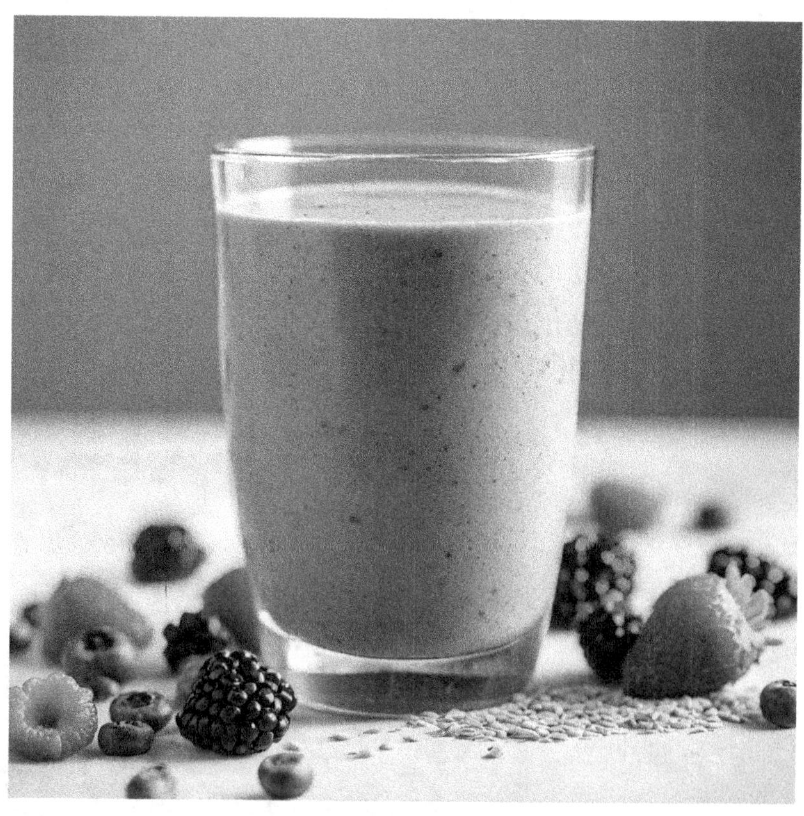

12. Steel-Cut Oats with Pumpkin Seeds and Dried Cranberries

Ingredients:

- 1 cup steel-cut oats
- 4 cups water
- 1/4 cup pumpkin seeds
- 1/4 cup dried cranberries
- 1/4 tsp cinnamon
- 1 tbsp honey or maple syrup

Instructions:

1. Bring water to a boil in a saucepan. Add oats and reduce heat to a simmer.
2. Cook uncovered, stirring occasionally, for about 20-30 minutes until oats are tender.
3. Stir in cinnamon, pumpkin seeds, and dried cranberries. Sweeten with honey or maple syrup.
4. Serve warm.

Nutrition Info Per Serving (Serves 4):

- Calories: 230
- Fat: 6g
- Carbohydrates: 39g
- Protein: 8g
- Sodium: 10mg

Cooking Time:

- Preparation time: 5 minutes
- Cooking time: 30 minutes
- Total time: 35 minutes

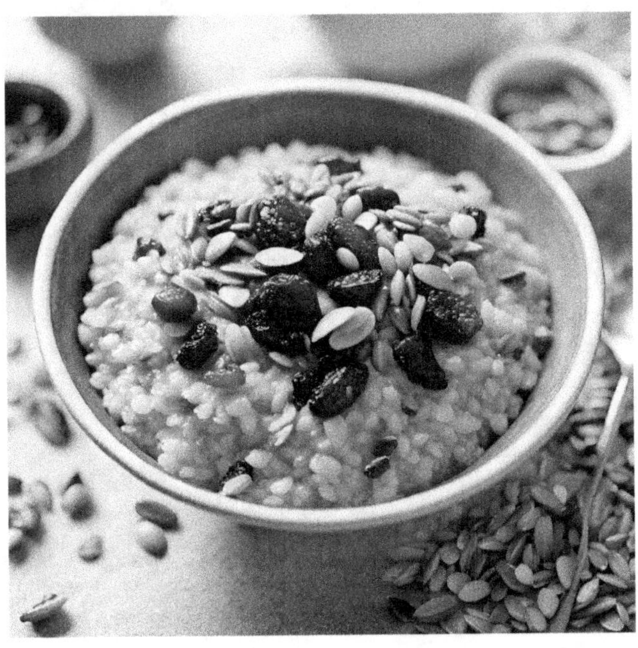

13. Pear and Ginger Compote on Ricotta Toast

Ingredients:

- 2 pears, peeled and chopped
- 1 tsp grated ginger
- 1/4 cup water
- 1 tbsp honey
- 4 slices whole wheat bread
- 1 cup ricotta cheese

Instructions:

1. In a small saucepan, combine pears, ginger, water, and honey. Simmer over medium heat until pears are soft and the mixture has thickened, about 10 minutes.
2. Toast the bread slices.
3. Spread ricotta on each slice of toast.
4. Top with pear and ginger compote.
5. Serve immediately.

Nutrition Info Per Serving (Serves 4):

- Calories: 250
- Fat: 8g
- Carbohydrates: 36g
- Protein: 10g
- Sodium: 180mg

Cooking Time:

- Preparation time: 10 minutes
- Cooking time: 10 minutes
- Total time: 20 minutes

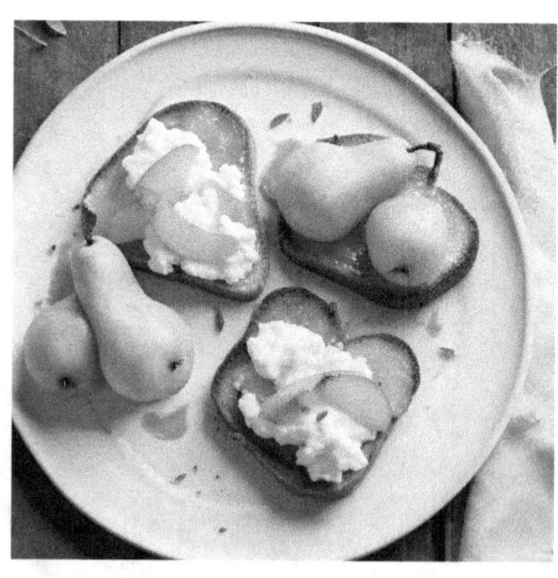

14. Kale and White Bean Breakfast Hash

Ingredients:

- 1 tbsp olive oil
- 1 onion, diced
- 2 cloves garlic, minced
- 2 cups chopped kale
- 1 cup cooked white beans
- 1 red bell pepper, diced
- Salt and pepper to taste
- 1/4 tsp smoked paprika

Instructions:

1. Heat olive oil in a large skillet over medium heat.
2. Add onion and garlic; sauté until onion is translucent.
3. Add bell pepper and cook for another 5 minutes.
4. Stir in kale and cook until wilted, about 3 minutes.
5. Mix in white beans, smoked paprika, salt, and pepper; cook until beans are heated through, about 5 minutes.
6. Serve hot.

Nutrition Info Per Serving (Serves 4):

- Calories: 160
- Fat: 4g
- Carbohydrates: 25g
- Protein: 8g
- Sodium: 300mg

Cooking Time:

- Preparation time: 10 minutes
- Cooking time: 20 minutes
- Total time: 30 minutes

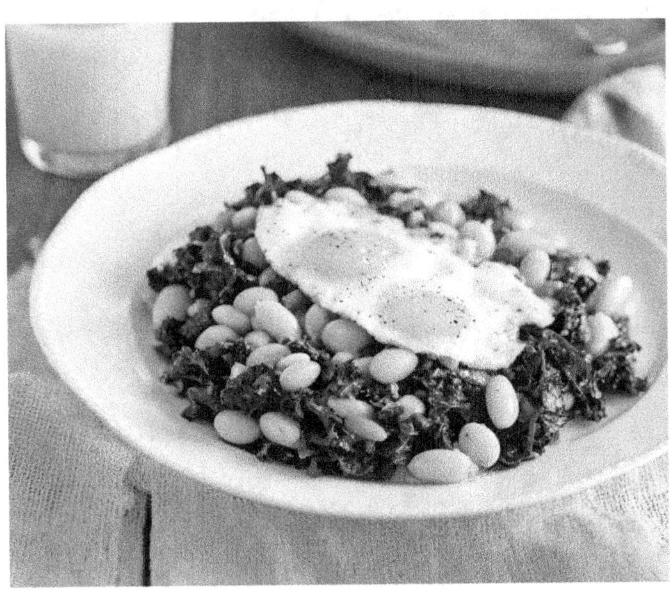

15. Apple Cinnamon Bran Muffins

Ingredients:

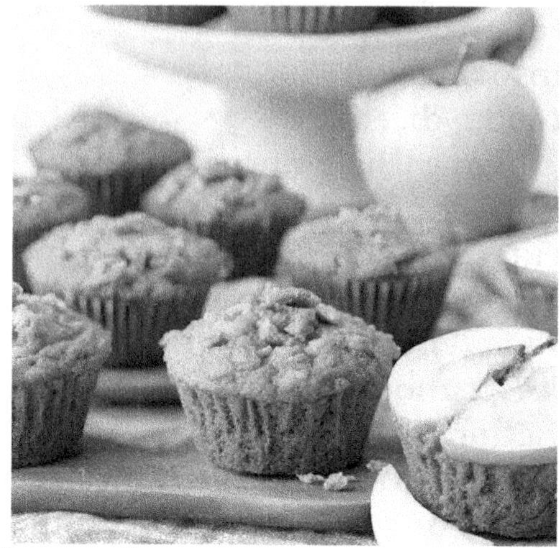

- 1½ cups wheat bran
- 1 cup whole wheat flour
- 1½ tsp baking powder
- 1 tsp baking soda
- 1 tsp cinnamon
- ½ tsp salt
- 1 egg
- ⅓ cup honey
- 1 cup buttermilk
- ⅓ cup vegetable oil
- 1 tsp vanilla extract
- 1 large apple, peeled, cored, and chopped

Instructions:

1. Preheat the oven to 375°F (190°C). Line a muffin tin with paper liners.
2. In a large bowl, mix together wheat bran, whole wheat flour, baking powder, baking soda, cinnamon, and salt.
3. In another bowl, whisk together the egg, honey, buttermilk, oil, and vanilla extract.
4. Stir the wet ingredients into the dry ingredients until just combined. Fold in the chopped apple.
5. Spoon the batter into the muffin tin, filling each cup about three-quarters full.
6. Bake for 15-20 minutes, or until a toothpick inserted into the center of a muffin comes out clean.
7. Allow muffins to cool in the pan for 5 minutes, then transfer to a wire rack to cool completely.

Nutrition Info Per Serving (Serves 12):

- Calories: 180
- Fat: 7g
- Carbohydrates: 28g
- Protein: 4g
- Sodium: 210mg

Cooking Time:

- Preparation time: 10 minutes
- Cooking time: 20 minutes
- Total time: 30 minutes

16. Rye Bread Avocado Toast with Tomato Slices

Ingredients:

- 4 slices rye bread
- 2 ripe avocados, mashed
- 1 large tomato, sliced
- Salt and pepper to taste
- Red pepper flakes (optional)

Instructions:

1. Toast the rye bread slices until crisp and golden.
2. Spread the mashed avocado evenly over each slice of toast.
3. Top with sliced tomatoes and season with salt, pepper, and red pepper flakes if using.
4. Serve immediately.

Nutrition Info Per Serving (Serves 4):

- Calories: 250
- Fat: 15g
- Carbohydrates: 27g
- Protein: 6g
- Sodium: 300mg

Cooking Time:

- Preparation time: 5 minutes
- Total time: 5 minutes

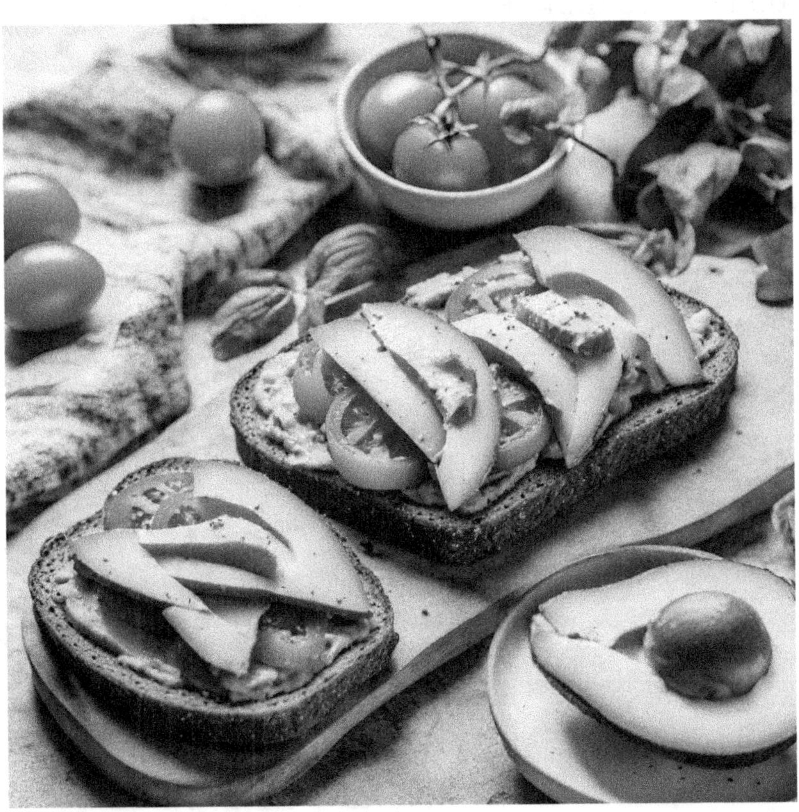

17. Muesli with Skim Milk and Dried Fruit

Ingredients:

- 2 cups rolled oats
- ¼ cup wheat germ
- ¼ cup sunflower seeds
- ¼ cup chopped almonds
- ¼ cup dried cranberries
- ¼ cup raisins
- 4 cups skim milk

Instructions:

1. In a large bowl, mix together the oats, wheat germ, sunflower seeds, almonds, dried cranberries, and raisins.
2. Divide the mixture into bowls and pour skim milk over each serving.
3. Serve immediately, or for best results, let sit in the refrigerator overnight to soften the grains.

Nutrition Info Per Serving (Serves 4):

- Calories: 350
- Fat: 10g
- Carbohydrates: 53g
- Protein: 17g
- Sodium: 120mg

Cooking Time:

- Preparation time: 5 minutes
- Total time: 5 minutes

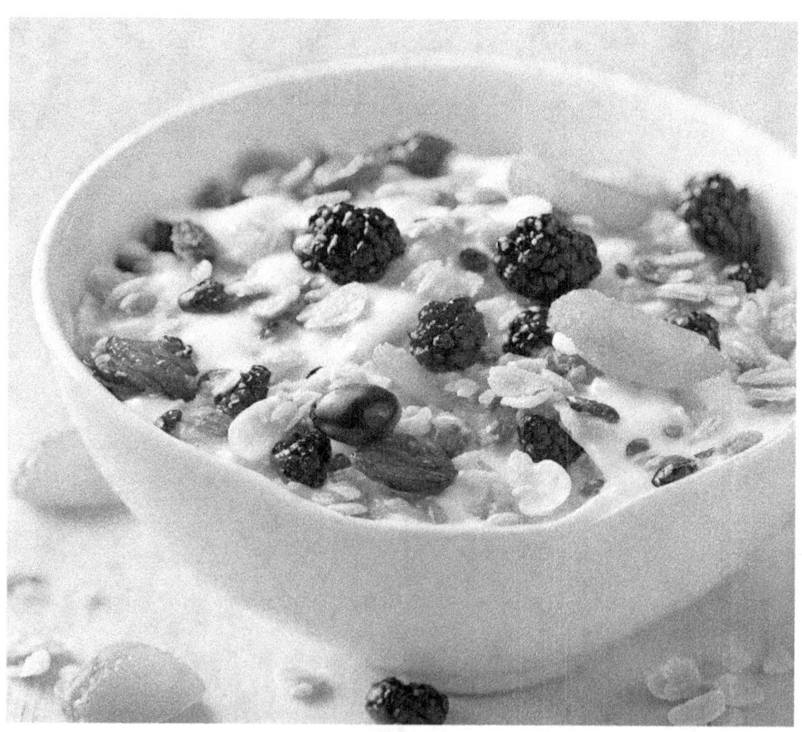

18. Spelt Waffles with Fresh Berries

Ingredients:

- 2 cups spelt flour
- 2 tsp baking powder
- ½ tsp salt
- 2 eggs, beaten
- 1½ cups milk
- ⅓ cup vegetable oil
- 2 cups mixed fresh berries (blueberries, raspberries, strawberries)

Instructions:

1. Preheat a waffle iron according to manufacturer's instructions.
2. In a bowl, whisk together spelt flour, baking powder, and salt.
3. In another bowl, mix the eggs, milk, and oil. Stir into the dry ingredients until just combined.
4. Pour batter onto the hot waffle iron and cook until golden and crisp.
5. Serve hot waffles topped with fresh berries.

Nutrition Info Per Serving (Serves 4):

- Calories: 440
- Fat: 23g
- Carbohydrates: 49g
- Protein: 13g
- Sodium: 380mg

Cooking Time:

- Preparation time: 10 minutes
- Cooking time: 10 minutes
- Total time: 20 minutes

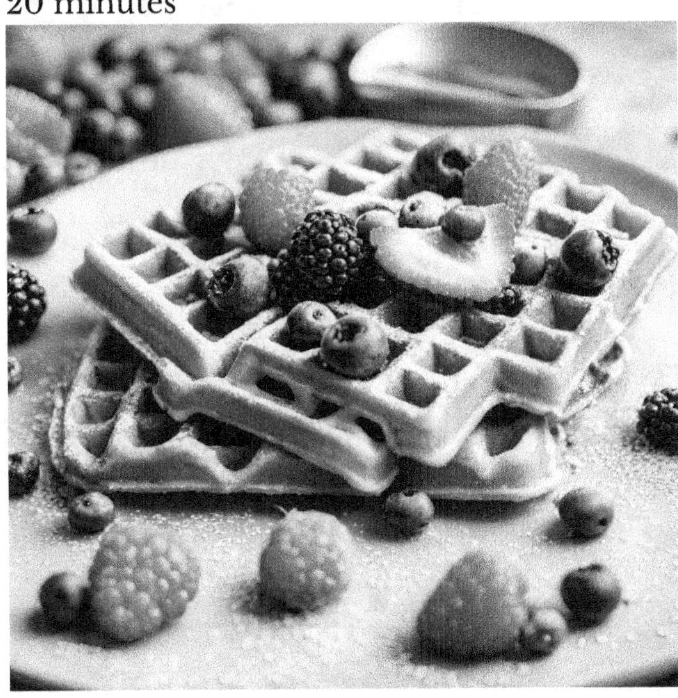

19. Overnight Oats with Chia Seeds and Peach
Ingredients:
- 1 cup rolled oats
- 2 tbsp chia seeds
- 1 cup almond milk
- 1 peach, diced
- 1 tbsp honey or maple syrup

Instructions:
1. In a jar or bowl, combine the oats, chia seeds, and almond milk.
2. Stir in the diced peach and sweeten with honey or maple syrup.
3. Cover and refrigerate overnight.
4. Serve chilled, stirred well.

Nutrition Info Per Serving (Serves 2):
- Calories: 290
- Fat: 9g
- Carbohydrates: 45g
- Protein: 9g
- Sodium: 80mg

Cooking Time:
- Preparation time: 5 minutes
- Total time: Overnight (at least 8 hours)

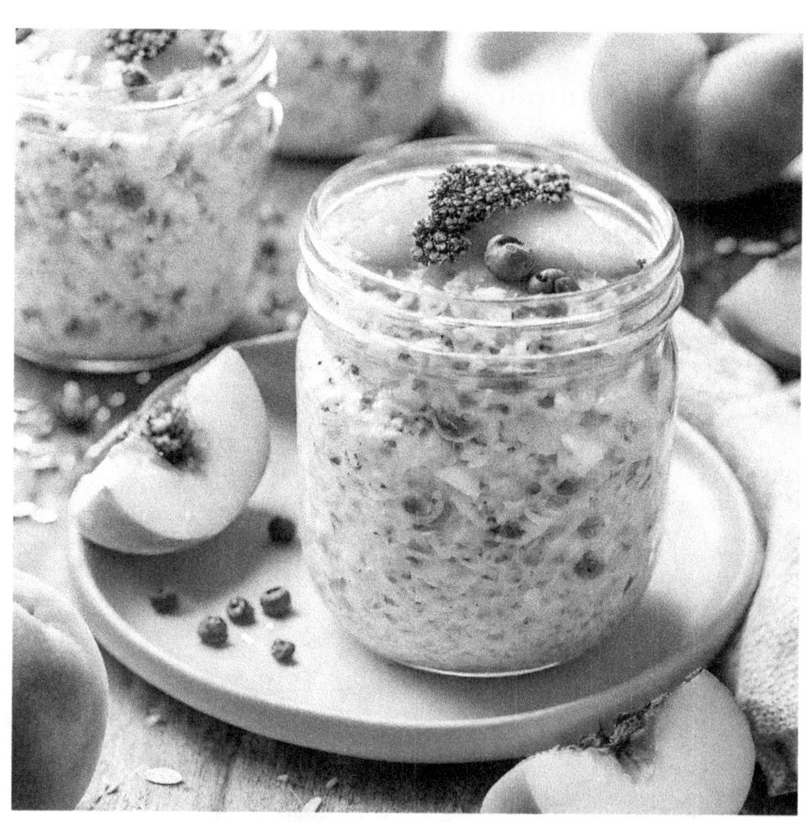

20. Baked Sweet Potato and Poached Eggs

Ingredients:

- 2 large sweet potatoes, scrubbed and pierced with a fork
- 4 eggs
- Salt and pepper to taste
- Fresh herbs (such as parsley or chives), for garnish

Instructions:

1. Preheat the oven to 400°F (200°C). Place the sweet potatoes on a baking sheet and bake until tender, about 45 minutes.
2. About 10 minutes before the sweet potatoes are done, poach the eggs. Fill a saucepan with water, bring to a simmer, and add a little vinegar. Crack each egg into a cup and gently pour into the simmering water. Poach for about 3-4 minutes or until the whites are set.
3. Split the baked sweet potatoes open and place each on a plate. Top each with a poached egg.
4. Season with salt and pepper, and garnish with fresh herbs.

Nutrition Info Per Serving (Serves 4):

- Calories: 200
- Fat: 5g
- Carbohydrates: 30g
- Protein: 8g
- Sodium: 150mg

Cooking Time:

- Preparation time: 5 minutes
- Cooking time: 45 minutes
- Total time: 50 minutes

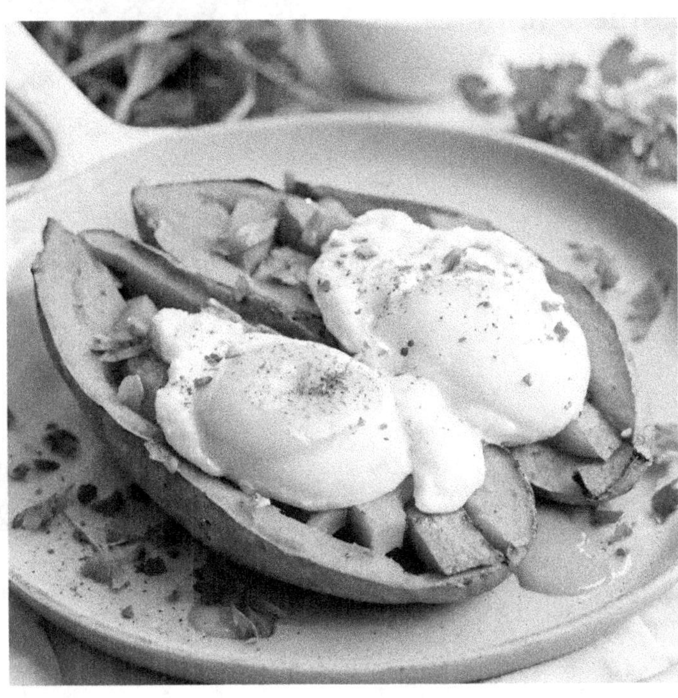

21. Barley Porridge with Dates and Cardamom

Ingredients:

- 1 cup hulled barley, rinsed
- 4 cups water
- 1/2 tsp salt
- 1/2 cup chopped dates
- 1/2 tsp ground cardamom
- 1/4 cup milk (almond or cow's milk)
- 1 tbsp honey or maple syrup

Instructions:

1. In a medium saucepan, combine barley, water, and salt. Bring to a boil over high heat.
2. Reduce heat to low, cover, and simmer for about 45 minutes, or until barley is tender and most of the water is absorbed.
3. Stir in chopped dates and cardamom, and continue to cook for 5 more minutes.
4. Add milk and honey (or maple syrup), stir well, and heat through for another minute.
5. Serve hot, with additional milk if desired.

Nutrition Info Per Serving (Serves 4):

- Calories: 220
- Fat: 1g
- Carbohydrates: 48g
- Protein: 5g
- Sodium: 300mg

Cooking Time:

- Preparation time: 5 minutes
- Cooking time: 50 minutes
- Total time: 55 minutes

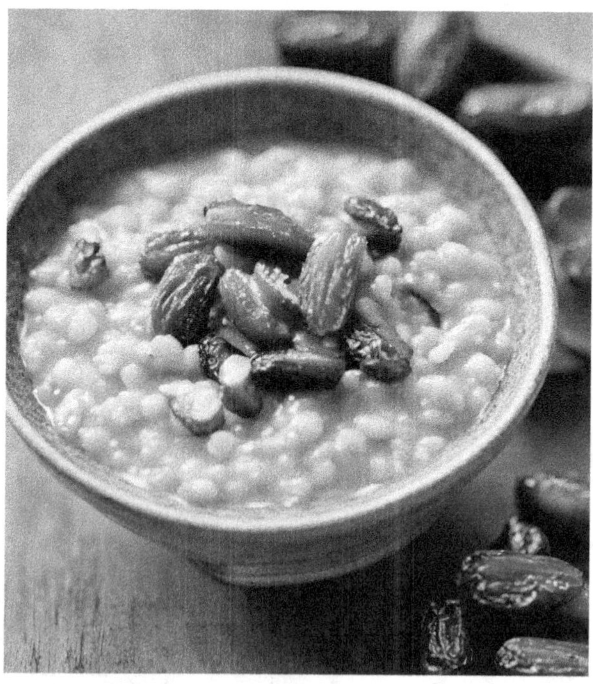

22. Banana and Walnut Muffins (made with almond flour)

Ingredients:

- 2 cups almond flour
- 1 tsp baking soda
- 1/4 tsp salt
- 3 ripe bananas, mashed
- 3 eggs
- 1/4 cup honey
- 1/4 cup vegetable oil
- 1 tsp vanilla extract
- 1/2 cup walnuts, chopped

Instructions:

1. Preheat the oven to 350°F (175°C). Line a muffin tin with paper liners or grease with oil.
2. In a bowl, mix together almond flour, baking soda, and salt.
3. In another bowl, whisk together mashed bananas, eggs, honey, oil, and vanilla extract.
4. Add the wet ingredients to the dry ingredients and stir until combined. Fold in chopped walnuts.
5. Divide the batter evenly among the muffin cups.
6. Bake for 20-25 minutes, or until a toothpick inserted into the center of a muffin comes out clean.
7. Allow to cool in the pan for 10 minutes, then transfer to a wire rack to cool completely.

Nutrition Info Per Serving (Makes 12 muffins):

- Calories: 240
- Fat: 16g
- Carbohydrates: 20g
- Protein: 7g
- Sodium: 210mg

Cooking Time:

- Preparation time: 10 minutes
- Cooking time: 25 minutes
- Total time: 35 minutes

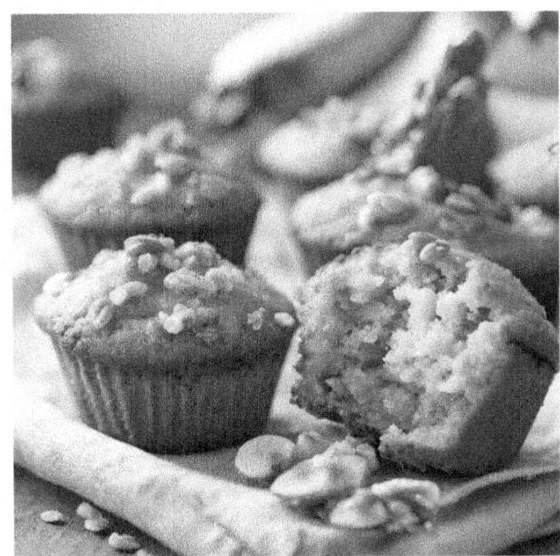

23. Greek Yogurt with Flaxseeds and Honey

Ingredients:

- 2 cups Greek yogurt
- 2 tbsp ground flaxseeds
- 2 tbsp honey
- Fresh fruit for topping (optional)

Instructions:

1. In a bowl, mix together Greek yogurt, ground flaxseeds, and honey.
2. Divide the yogurt mixture into servings and top with fresh fruit if desired.
3. Serve immediately or chill in the refrigerator until ready to eat.

Nutrition Info Per Serving (Serves 2):

- Calories: 290
- Fat: 9g
- Carbohydrates: 36g
- Protein: 20g
- Sodium: 70mg

Cooking Time:

- Preparation time: 5 minutes
- Total time: 5 minutes

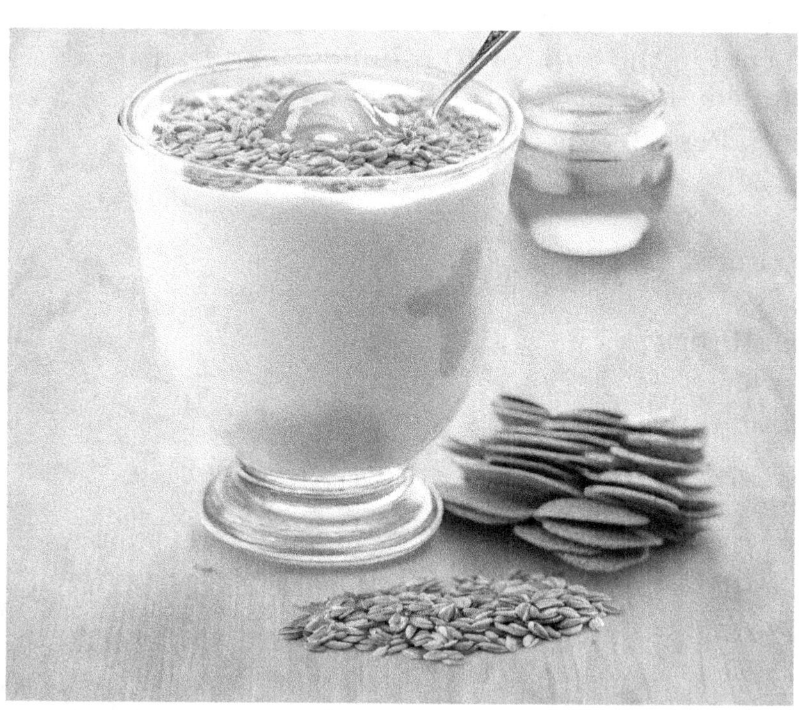

24. Vegetable Omelette with Spinach and Mushrooms

Ingredients:

- 4 eggs
- 1/2 cup chopped spinach
- 1/2 cup sliced mushrooms
- 1/4 cup diced onions
- 1 clove garlic, minced
- 2 tbsp olive oil
- Salt and pepper to taste

Instructions:

1. Heat olive oil in a skillet over medium heat. Add onions and garlic, sauté until translucent.
2. Add mushrooms and spinach, cook until the spinach is wilted and mushrooms are golden.
3. In a bowl, whisk the eggs with salt and pepper.
4. Pour the eggs over the vegetables in the skillet. Cook until the eggs are set, about 4-5 minutes.
5. Fold the omelette in half and serve hot.

Nutrition Info Per Serving (Serves 2):

- Calories: 300
- Fat: 23g
- Carbohydrates: 7g
- Protein: 16g
- Sodium: 170mg

Cooking Time:

- Preparation time: 10 minutes
- Cooking time: 10 minutes
- Total time: 20 minutes

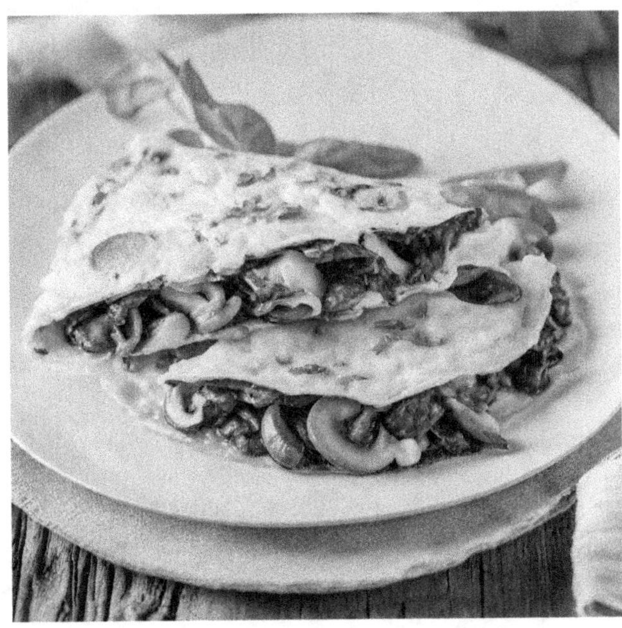

25. Buckwheat Pancakes with Maple Syrup

Ingredients:

- 1 cup buckwheat flour
- 1 tsp baking powder
- 1/4 tsp salt
- 1 egg
- 1 cup milk (any kind)
- 2 tbsp melted butter or oil
- Maple syrup for serving
- Fresh berries for serving

Instructions:

1. In a bowl, mix together buckwheat flour, baking powder, and salt.
2. In another bowl, whisk together egg, milk, and melted butter or oil.
3. Stir the wet ingredients into the dry ingredients until just combined.
4. Heat a non-stick skillet over medium heat. Pour 1/4 cup of batter for each pancake and cook until bubbles form on the surface, then flip and cook until golden brown on the other side.
5. Serve hot with maple syrup and fresh berries.

Nutrition Info Per Serving (Serves 4):

- Calories: 220
- Fat: 9g
- Carbohydrates: 30g
- Protein: 6g
- Sodium: 320mg

Cooking Time:

- Preparation time: 10 minutes
- Cooking time: 10 minutes
- Total time: 20 minutes

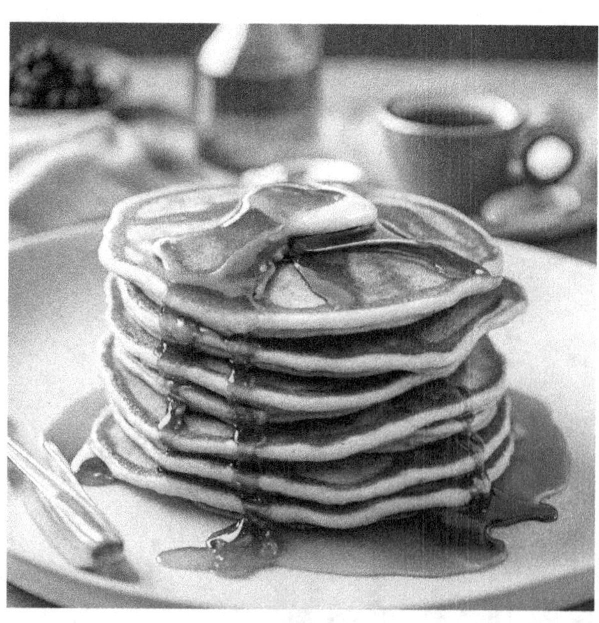

Poultry & Meat Recipes

1. Grilled Chicken with Herbs and Lemon

Ingredients:

- 4 boneless, skinless chicken breasts
- 2 lemons, juiced and zested
- 2 cloves garlic, minced
- 1 tbsp fresh rosemary, chopped
- 1 tbsp fresh thyme, chopped
- 2 tbsp olive oil
- Salt and pepper to taste

Instructions:

1. In a bowl, mix together lemon juice, lemon zest, minced garlic, rosemary, thyme, olive oil, salt, and pepper.
2. Place chicken breasts in a resealable plastic bag or shallow dish. Pour the marinade over the chicken, making sure it's well-coated. Refrigerate for at least 1 hour, or overnight for more flavor.
3. Preheat grill to medium-high heat.
4. Remove chicken from marinade and grill for 6-7 minutes on each side, or until the internal temperature reaches 165°F (75°C).
5. Let the chicken rest for a few minutes before serving.

Nutrition Info Per Serving (Serves 4):

- Calories: 220
- Fat: 10g
- Carbohydrates: 3g
- Protein: 29g
- Sodium: 150mg

Cooking Time:

- Preparation time: 10 minutes (plus marinating time)
- Cooking time: 15 minutes
- Total time: 25 minutes (plus marinating time)

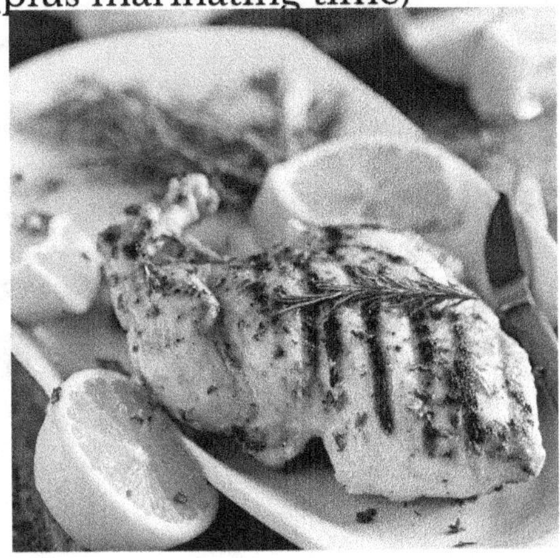

2. Turkey and Quinoa Stuffed Peppers

Ingredients:

- 4 large bell peppers, tops cut off and seeded
- 1 lb ground turkey
- 1 cup cooked quinoa
- 1 onion, chopped
- 1 zucchini, diced
- 1 cup spinach, chopped
- 2 cloves garlic, minced
- 1 cup tomato sauce
- 1 tsp dried oregano
- 1 tsp dried basil
- Salt and pepper to taste
- 1/2 cup shredded mozzarella cheese (optional)

Instructions:

1. Preheat oven to 375°F (190°C).
2. In a skillet over medium heat, cook the ground turkey until browned. Add onion, zucchini, and garlic, cooking until vegetables are soft.
3. Stir in cooked quinoa, spinach, tomato sauce, oregano, basil, salt, and pepper. Cook until the mixture is heated through and spinach is wilted.
4. Stuff the bell peppers with the turkey and quinoa mixture. Place in a baking dish.
5. Top with mozzarella cheese if using. Cover with aluminum foil.
6. Bake in the preheated oven for 30 minutes. Remove the foil and bake for an additional 10 minutes or until the peppers are tender and the cheese is bubbly.

Nutrition Info Per Serving (Serves 4):

- Calories: 350
- Fat: 14g
- Carbohydrates: 33g
- Protein: 27g
- Sodium: 400mg

Cooking Time:

- Preparation time: 20 minutes
- Cooking time: 40 minutes
- Total time: 60 minutes

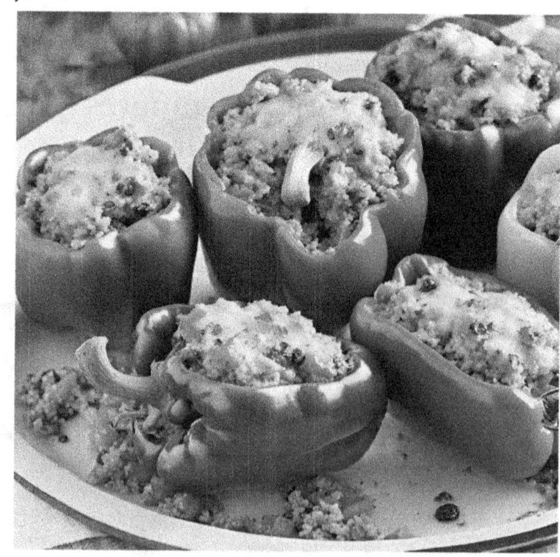

3. Beef and Broccoli Stir-Fry

Ingredients:

- 1 lb beef sirloin, thinly sliced
- 4 cups broccoli florets
- 2 tbsp vegetable oil
- 2 cloves garlic, minced
- 1 tbsp ginger, minced
- 1/4 cup soy sauce (low sodium)
- 1 tbsp oyster sauce
- 1 tbsp cornstarch
- 1/2 cup water
- 1 tsp sesame oil

Instructions:

1. In a small bowl, mix the soy sauce, oyster sauce, cornstarch, water, and sesame oil to make the sauce.
2. Heat vegetable oil in a large skillet or wok over medium-high heat. Add garlic and ginger, sautéing until fragrant.
3. Add the beef and cook until it starts to brown, about 3-4 minutes.
4. Add broccoli and stir-fry for another 5 minutes, or until the broccoli is tender but still crisp.
5. Pour the sauce over the beef and broccoli, mixing well. Cook for another 2-3 minutes until the sauce has thickened.
6. Serve hot with rice or noodles.

Nutrition Info Per Serving (Serves 4):

- Calories: 280
- Fat: 15g
- Carbohydrates: 13g
- Protein: 26g
- Sodium: 600mg

Cooking Time:

- Preparation time: 10 minutes
- Cooking time: 15 minutes
- Total time: 25 minutes

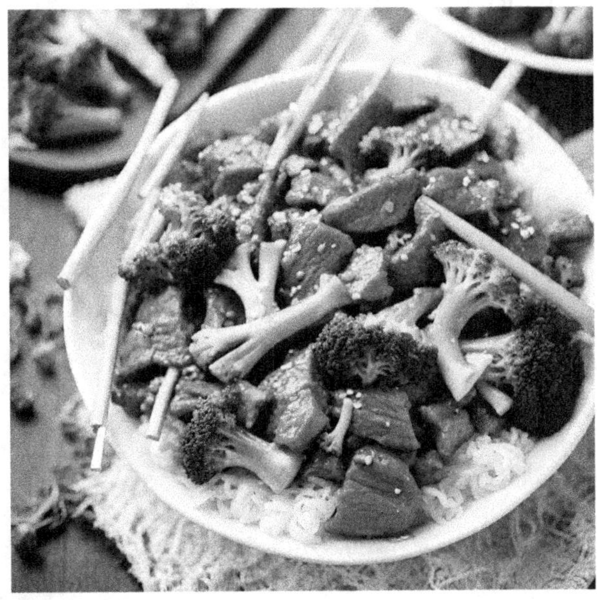

4. Balsamic Glazed Chicken Breast

Ingredients:

- 4 boneless, skinless chicken breasts
- 1/4 cup balsamic vinegar
- 2 tbsp honey
- 2 cloves garlic, minced
- 1 tbsp olive oil
- Salt and pepper to taste

Instructions:

1. Preheat the oven to 400°F (200°C).
2. In a small saucepan, combine balsamic vinegar, honey, and minced garlic. Bring to a boil, then reduce heat and simmer until the mixture thickens into a glaze, about 10 minutes , stirring occasionally.
3. Heat olive oil in a skillet over medium-high heat. Season the chicken breasts with salt and pepper.
4. Sear the chicken in the skillet for about 3 minutes on each side until golden brown.
5. Transfer the chicken to a baking dish and brush with the balsamic glaze.
6. Bake in the preheated oven for 15-20 minutes, or until the chicken is cooked through and the internal temperature reaches 165°F (75°C).
7. Baste the chicken with the remaining glaze halfway through cooking.
8. Serve the chicken sliced, with extra glaze drizzled on top.

Nutrition Info Per Serving (Serves 4):

- Calories: 240
- Fat: 7g
- Carbohydrates: 12g
- Protein: 30g
- Sodium: 220mg

Cooking Time:

- Preparation time: 10 minutes
- Cooking time: 30 minutes
- Total time: 40 minutes

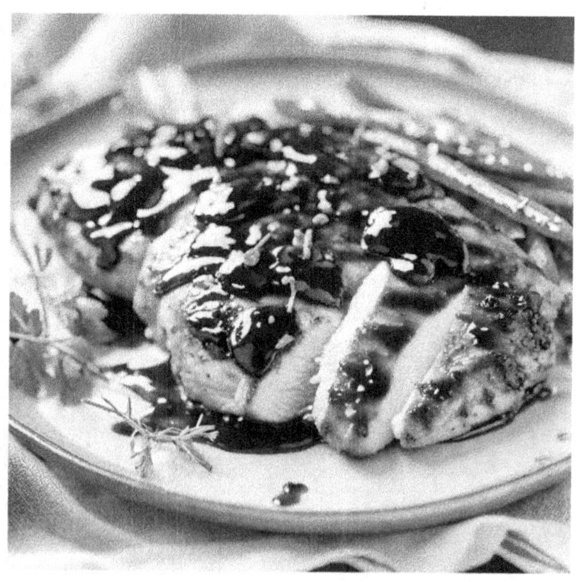

5. Lamb Tagine with Apricots

Ingredients:

- 2 lbs lamb shoulder, cut into 1-inch cubes
- 1 onion, chopped
- 2 cloves garlic, minced
- 1 tsp ground cumin
- 1 tsp ground coriander
- 1/2 tsp cinnamon
- 2 cups beef or vegetable broth
- 1 cup dried apricots, halved
- 1/2 cup almonds, toasted
- 2 tbsp olive oil
- Salt and pepper to taste
- Fresh cilantro, chopped (for garnish)

Instructions:

1. Heat olive oil in a tagine or large pot over medium heat. Add the lamb cubes and brown on all sides. Remove and set aside.
2. In the same pot, add onions and garlic, cooking until softened.
3. Return the lamb to the pot and stir in cumin, coriander, and cinnamon.
4. Pour in broth and bring to a boil. Reduce heat to low, cover, and simmer for 1 hour.
5. Add dried apricots and continue to simmer for another 30 minutes, or until the lamb is tender.
6. Stir in toasted almonds and season with salt and pepper.
7. Garnish with chopped cilantro and serve.

Nutrition Info Per Serving (Serves 6):

- Calories: 460
- Fat: 28g
- Carbohydrates: 23g
- Protein: 34g
- Sodium: 300mg

Cooking Time:

- Preparation time: 15 minutes
- Cooking time: 1 hour 45 minutes
- Total time: 2 hours

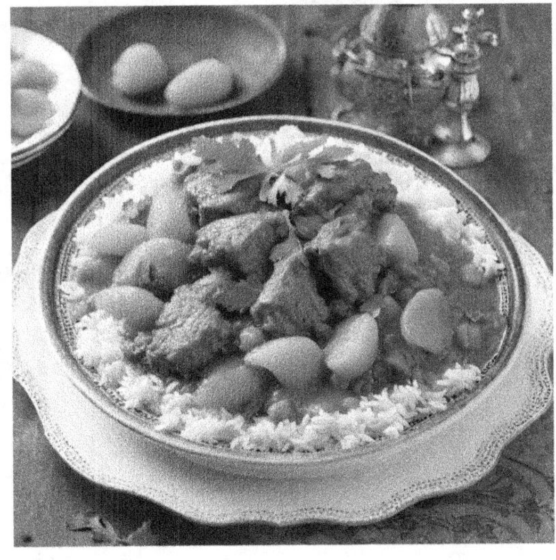

6. Pork Tenderloin with Roasted Apples and Onions

Ingredients:

- 2 lbs pork tenderloin
- 2 apples, sliced
- 2 onions, sliced
- 1/4 cup apple cider vinegar
- 1/4 cup olive oil
- 2 tbsp honey
- 1 tsp thyme
- Salt and pepper to taste

Instructions:

1. Preheat the oven to 375°F (190°C).
2. Place the sliced apples and onions in a roasting pan.
3. In a small bowl, mix together apple cider vinegar, olive oil, honey, and thyme.
4. Season the pork tenderloin with salt and pepper and place it on top of the apples and onions.
5. Pour the vinegar mixture over the pork.
6. Roast in the preheated oven for 25-30 minutes, or until the pork reaches an internal temperature of 145°F (63°C).
7. Let the pork rest for 5 minutes before slicing. Serve with the roasted apples and onions.

Nutrition Info Per Serving (Serves 4):

- Calories: 410
- Fat: 18g
- Carbohydrates: 27g
- Protein: 36g
- Sodium: 200mg

Cooking Time:

- Preparation time: 10 minutes
- Cooking time: 30 minutes
- Total time: 40 minutes

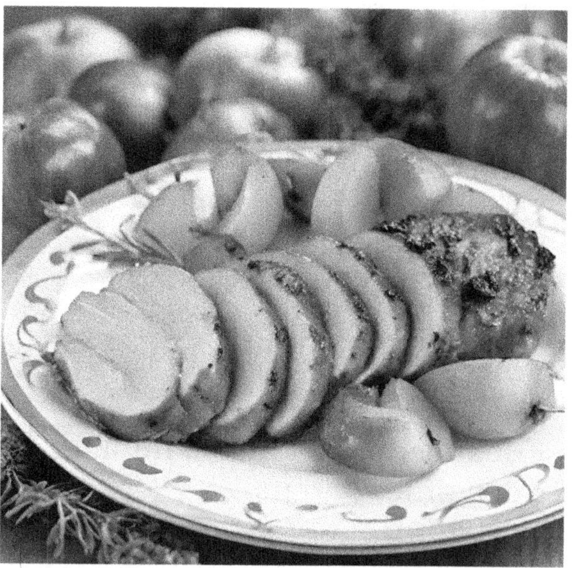

7. Chicken Caesar Salad

Ingredients:

- 2 boneless, skinless chicken breasts, grilled and sliced
- 6 cups Romaine lettuce, chopped
- 1/2 cup Parmesan cheese, grated
- 1 cup croutons
- Caesar dressing (preferably homemade or a low-fat store-bought version)
- 1 tsp olive oil
- Salt and pepper to taste
- Lemon wedges (for serving)

Instructions:

1. In a large salad bowl, combine chopped Romaine lettuce, Parmesan cheese, and croutons.
2. In a skillet, heat olive oil over medium heat. Season the chicken breasts with salt and pepper and grill until cooked through, about 6-7 minutes per side. Let cool and slice.
3. Add the grilled chicken to the salad.
4. Drizzle Caesar dressing over the salad and toss to coat evenly.
5. Serve with lemon wedges on the side.

Nutrition Info Per Serving (Serves 4):

- Calories: 320
- Fat: 16g
- Carbohydrates: 12g
- Protein: 30g
- Sodium: 400mg

Cooking Time:

- Preparation time: 15 minutes
- Cooking time: 15 minutes
- Total time: 30 minutes

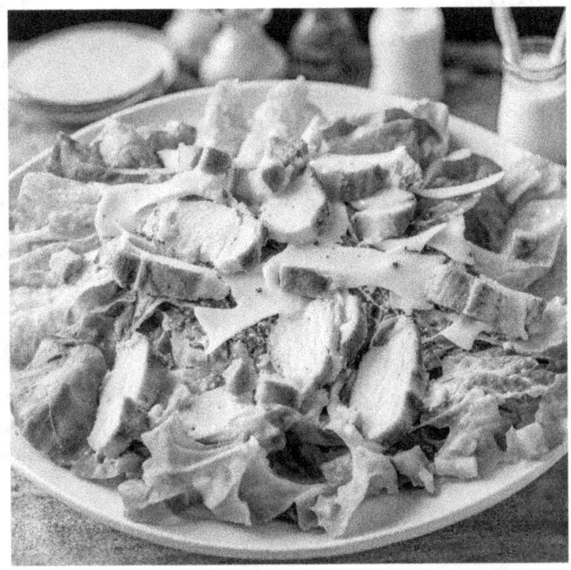

8. Beef Stew with Root Vegetables

Ingredients:

- 2 lbs beef chuck, cut into 1-inch cubes
- 3 carrots, peeled and chopped
- 2 parsnips, peeled and chopped
- 2 turnips, peeled and chopped
- 1 onion, chopped
- 3 cloves garlic, minced
- 4 cups beef broth
- 1/4 cup tomato paste
- 2 tbsp Worcestershire sauce
- 1 tsp thyme
- 2 tbsp olive oil
- Salt and pepper to taste

Instructions:

1. In a large pot, heat olive oil over medium-high heat. Add beef cubes and brown on all sides. Remove and set aside.
2. In the same pot, add onions and garlic, cooking until softened.
3. Return the beef to the pot along with carrots, parsnips, turnips, beef broth, tomato paste, Worcestershire sauce, and thyme.
4. Bring to a boil, then reduce heat to low, cover, and simmer for 2 hours or until the beef is tender and the vegetables are cooked through.
5. Season with salt and pepper to taste.
6. Serve hot.

Nutrition Info Per Serving (Serves 6):

- Calories: 350
- Fat: 18g
- Carbohydrates: 18g
- Protein: 29g
- Sodium: 550mg

Cooking Time:

- Preparation time: 15 minutes
- Cooking time: 2 hours
- Total time: 2 hours 15 minutes

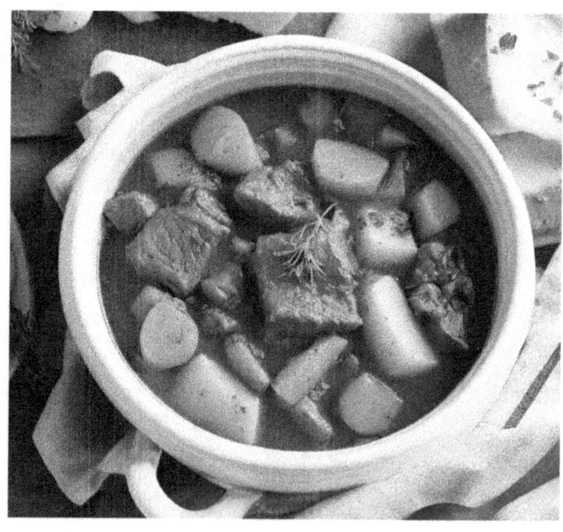

9. Spiced Turkey Burgers

Ingredients:

- 1 lb ground turkey
- 1 tsp cumin
- 1 tsp smoked paprika
- 1/2 tsp garlic powder
- 1/4 tsp salt
- 1/4 tsp black pepper
- 1 tbsp olive oil
- 4 whole wheat burger buns
- Lettuce, tomato slices, and onion slices for serving

Instructions:

1. In a bowl, mix together the ground turkey, cumin, smoked paprika, garlic powder, salt, and black pepper until well combined.
2. Form the mixture into 4 equal-sized patties.
3. Heat the olive oil in a skillet over medium heat. Cook the patties for about 5-6 minutes on each side, or until fully cooked and the internal temperature reaches 165°F (74°C).
4. Serve the patties on whole wheat buns with lettuce, tomato, and onion slices.

Nutrition Info Per Serving (Serves 4):

- Calories: 320
- Fat: 15g
- Carbohydrates: 23g
- Protein: 25g
- Sodium: 390mg

Cooking Time:

- Preparation time: 10 minutes
- Cooking time: 12 minutes
- Total time: 22 minutes

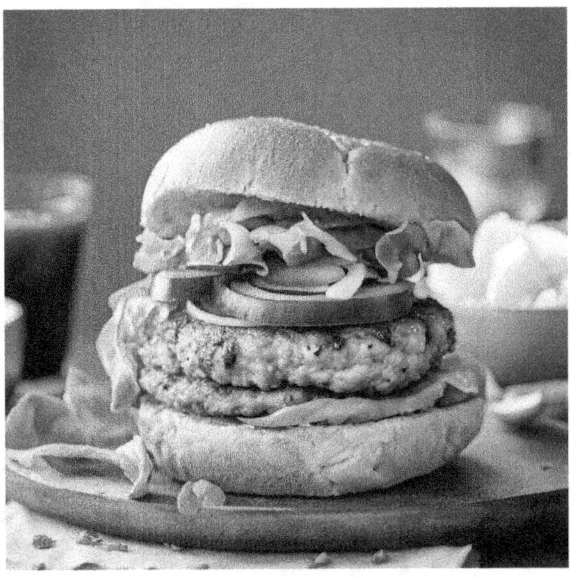

10. Chicken and Spinach Soup

Ingredients:

- 1 lb chicken breast, chopped
- 4 cups chicken broth
- 2 cups fresh spinach leaves
- 1 onion, diced
- 2 carrots, diced
- 2 stalks celery, diced
- 2 cloves garlic, minced
- 1 tsp thyme
- 1 tbsp olive oil
- Salt and pepper to taste

Instructions:

1. Heat olive oil in a large pot over medium heat. Add onion, carrots, celery, and garlic. Sauté until the vegetables are softened, about 5 minutes.
2. Add the chopped chicken breast and cook until no longer pink.
3. Pour in the chicken broth and bring to a boil. Reduce heat to a simmer and add thyme.
4. Simmer for 15 minutes, or until the chicken is fully cooked and the vegetables are tender.
5. Stir in the spinach and cook until wilted, about 2 minutes.
6. Season with salt and pepper to taste.
7. Serve hot.

Nutrition Info Per Serving (Serves 4):

- Calories: 180
- Fat: 5g
- Carbohydrates: 8g
- Protein: 25g
- Sodium: 870mg

Cooking Time:

- Preparation time: 10 minutes
- Cooking time: 25 minutes
- Total time: 35 minutes

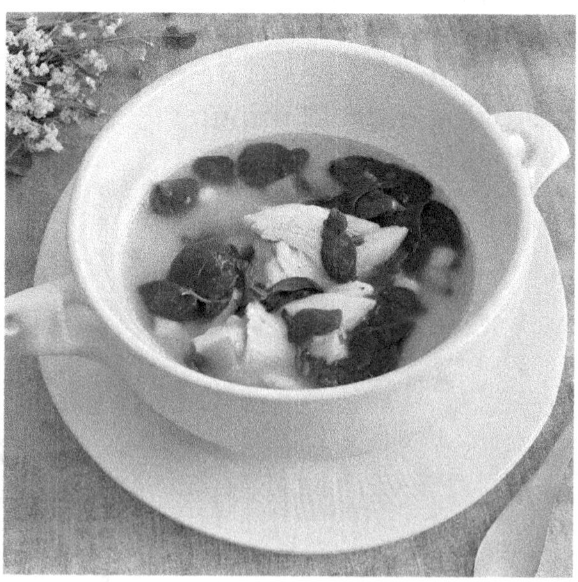

11. Roast Chicken with Garlic and Thyme

Ingredients:

- 1 whole chicken (about 4 lbs)
- 1 lemon, halved
- 4 cloves garlic, minced
- 2 tbsp fresh thyme, chopped
- 2 tbsp olive oil
- Salt and pepper to taste

Instructions:

1. Preheat the oven to 400°F (200°C).
2. Rub the chicken all over with olive oil, then season inside and out with salt, pepper, minced garlic, and thyme.
3. Place the lemon halves inside the cavity of the chicken.
4. Roast in the preheated oven for about 1 hour and 20 minutes, or until the chicken is cooked through and the skin is golden and crispy.
5. Let the chicken rest for 10 minutes before carving.
6. Serve with juices from the pan drizzled over the top.

Nutrition Info Per Serving (Serves 4):

- Calories: 410
- Fat: 30g
- Carbohydrates: 2g
- Protein: 32g
- Sodium: 380mg

Cooking Time:

- Preparation time: 10 minutes
- Cooking time: 1 hour 20 minutes
- Total time: 1 hour 30 minutes

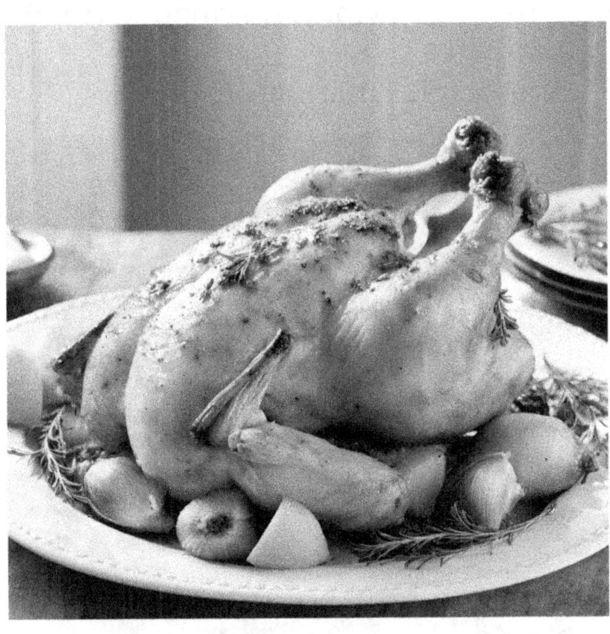

12. Beef Bulgogi

Ingredients:

- 1 lb thinly sliced beef sirloin
- 1/4 cup soy sauce (low sodium)
- 2 tbsp sesame oil
- 2 tbsp brown sugar
- 3 cloves garlic, minced
- 1 inch piece ginger, grated
- 2 green onions, chopped
- 1 tbsp sesame seeds
- 1 tsp black pepper

Instructions:

1. In a bowl, whisk together soy sauce, sesame oil, brown sugar, garlic, ginger, and black pepper to make the marinade.
2. Add the beef slices to the marinade, ensuring each piece is well-coated. Cover and refrigerate for at least 1 hour, or overnight for best flavor.
3. Heat a skillet or grill pan over high heat. Cook the marinated beef in batches, about 1-2 minutes per side, until browned and slightly caramelized.
4. Sprinkle with chopped green onions and sesame seeds before serving.
5. Serve hot with steamed rice or wrapped in lettuce leaves for a lighter option.

Nutrition Info Per Serving (Serves 4):

- Calories: 280 Fat: 15g Carbohydrates: 9g
- Protein: 27g
- Sodium: 590mg

Cooking Time:

- Preparation time: 10 minutes (plus marinating time)
- Cooking time: 10 minutes
- Total time: 20 minutes (plus marinating time)

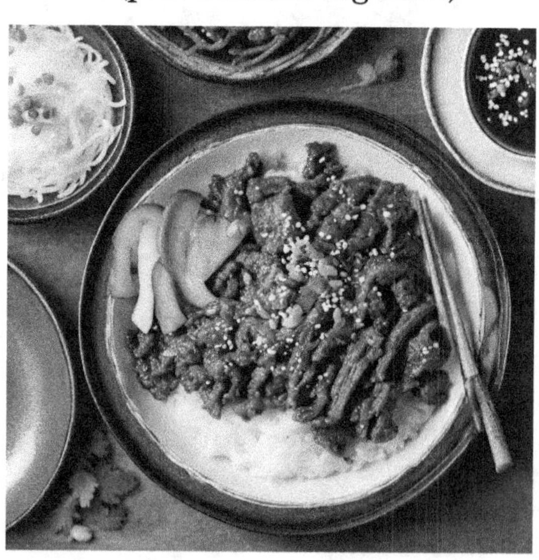

13. Moroccan Lamb with Squash and Dried Plums

Ingredients:

- 2 lbs lamb shoulder, cut into chunks
- 1 butternut squash, peeled and cubed
- 1 cup dried plums (prunes)
- 1 onion, chopped
- 3 cloves garlic, minced
- 1 tsp ground cinnamon
- 1 tsp ground cumin
- 1/2 tsp ground ginger
- 2 cups chicken or vegetable broth
- 2 tbsp olive oil
- Salt and pepper to taste
- Fresh cilantro, for garnish

Instructions:

1. Heat olive oil in a large pot over medium heat. Add the lamb chunks and brown on all sides. Remove and set aside.
2. In the same pot, add onion and garlic, cooking until softened.
3. Return the lamb to the pot along with the cinnamon, cumin, and ginger. Stir to coat the meat.
4. Add the broth, dried plums, and butternut squash. Bring to a boil, then reduce heat, cover, and simmer for 1.5 hours or until the lamb is tender.
5. Season with salt and pepper to taste.
6. Garnish with fresh cilantro before serving.

Nutrition Info Per Serving (Serves 6):

- Calories: 400
- Fat: 22g
- Carbohydrates: 30g
- Protein: 26g
- Sodium: 250mg

Cooking Time:

- Preparation time: 20 minutes
- Cooking time: 1 hour 50 minutes
- Total time: 2 hours 10 minutes

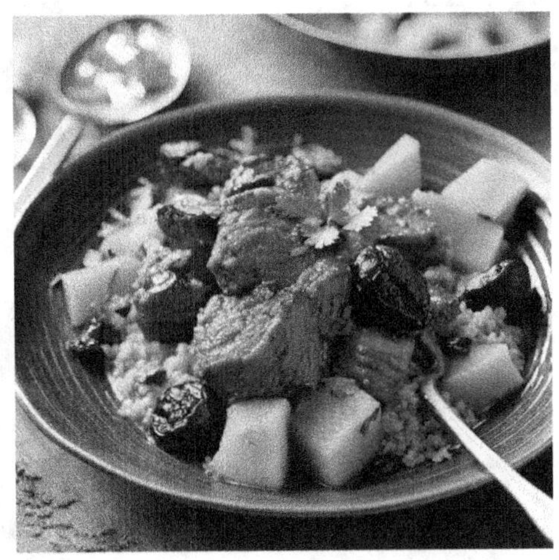

14. Pork Chops with Apple Cider Vinegar Sauce

Ingredients:

- 4 pork chops, bone-in
- 1 cup apple cider vinegar
- 2 tbsp honey
- 2 cloves garlic, minced
- 1 tbsp mustard
- 1 tbsp olive oil
- Salt and pepper to taste

Instructions:

1. Season pork chops with salt and pepper.
2. Heat olive oil in a skillet over medium-high heat. Add pork chops and sear until golden, about 5 minutes per side.
3. Remove chops from skillet and set aside.
4. In the same skillet, add garlic and sauté briefly.
5. Add apple cider vinegar, honey, and mustard. Stir to combine and bring to a simmer.
6. Return pork chops to the skillet, cover, and simmer for about 10 minutes, or until pork chops are cooked through.
7. Serve pork chops with the sauce drizzled over the top.

Nutrition Info Per Serving (Serves 4):

- Calories: 320
- Fat: 14g
- Carbohydrates: 12g
- Protein: 34g
- Sodium: 220mg

Cooking Time:

- Preparation time: 10 minutes
- Cooking time: 20 minutes
- Total time: 30 minutes

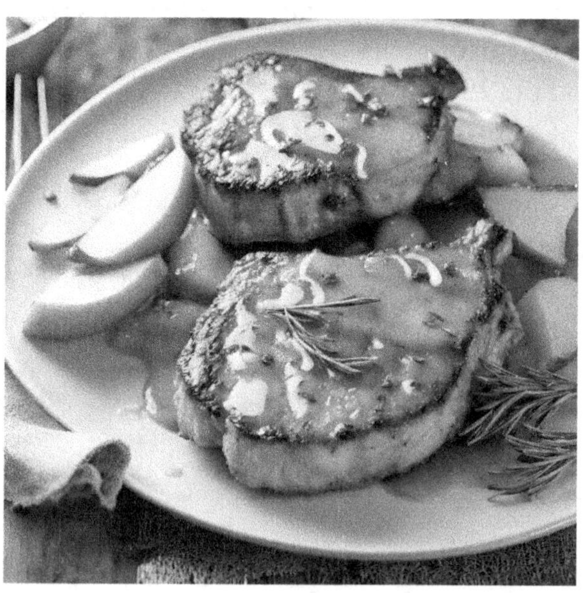

15. Chicken Tikka Masala

Ingredients:

- 2 lbs chicken breast, cubed
- 1 cup yogurt
- 2 tbsp lemon juice
- 2 tsp turmeric
- 2 tsp garam masala
- 1 tsp cumin
- 1 onion, chopped
- 3 cloves garlic, minced
- 1 can (28 oz) crushed tomatoes
- 1 cup cream
- 2 tbsp vegetable oil
- Salt to taste
- Fresh cilantro, for garnish

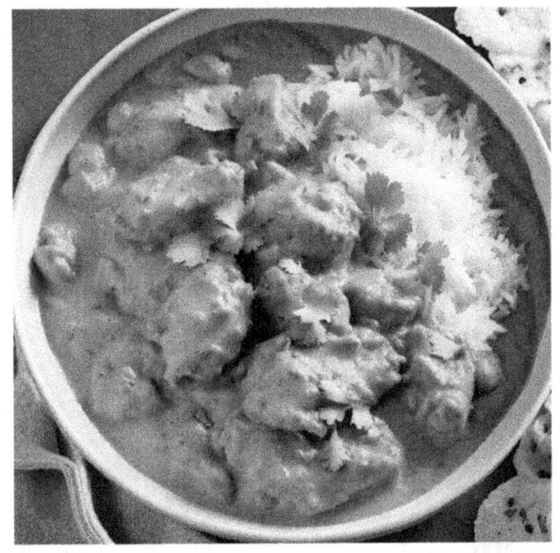

Instructions:

1. In a bowl, mix yogurt, lemon juice, turmeric, garam masala, and cumin. Add chicken, coat well, and marinate for at least 1 hour or overnight in the refrigerator.
2. Heat oil in a large skillet over medium heat. Add onion and garlic, and sauté until soft.
3. Add marinated chicken and cook until chicken is browned.
4. Add crushed tomatoes and bring to a simmer.
5. Reduce heat, add cream, and cook for another 10 minutes.
6. Season with salt and garnish with cilantro before serving.

Nutrition Info Per Serving (Serves 6):

- Calories: 460
- Fat: 28g
- Carbohydrates: 15g
- Protein: 37g
- Sodium: 200mg

Cooking Time:

- Preparation time: 15 minutes (plus marinating time)
- Cooking time: 30 minutes
- Total time: 45 minutes (plus marinating time)

16. Meatloaf with Oatmeal

Ingredients:

- 2 lbs ground beef
- 1 cup oatmeal
- 1 onion, finely chopped
- 2 cloves garlic, minced
- 1 egg
- 1/2 cup milk
- 2 tbsp ketchup
- 1 tbsp Worcestershire sauce
- Salt and pepper to taste
- 2 tbsp parsley, chopped (for garnish)

Instructions:

1. Preheat oven to 375°F (190°C).
2. In a large bowl, mix together all ingredients except parsley. Form into a loaf and place in a baking dish.
3. Bake in the preheated oven for 1 hour or until the meatloaf is cooked through.
4. Let stand for 10 minutes before slicing. Garnish with parsley.

Nutrition Info Per Serving (Serves 6):

- Calories: 380
- Fat: 22g
- Carbohydrates: 15g
- Protein: 30g
- Sodium: 250mg

Cooking Time:

- Preparation time: 15 minutes
- Cooking time: 1 hour
- Total time: 1 hour 15 minutes

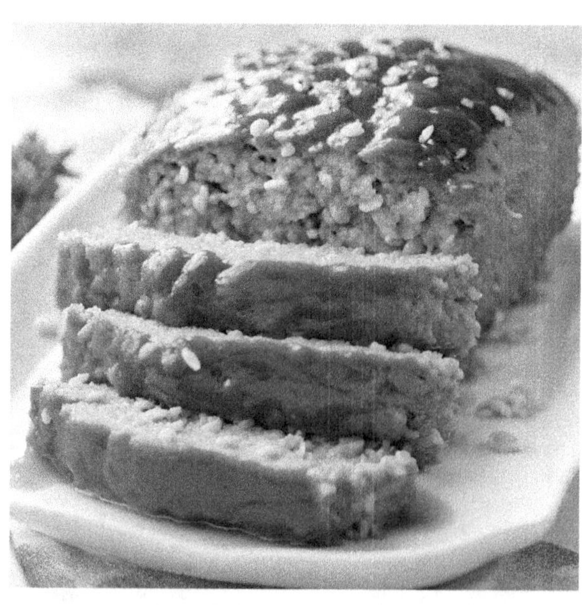

17. Duck Breast with Cherry Sauce

Ingredients:

- 2 duck breasts, skin scored
- 1 cup fresh or frozen cherries, pitted
- 1/4 cup red wine
- 1 tbsp balsamic vinegar
- 1 tbsp honey
- 1 tsp fresh thyme
- Salt and pepper to taste

Instructions:

1. Preheat oven to 400°F (200°C).
2. Season duck breasts with salt and pepper. Place them skin-side down in a cold skillet.
3. Turn heat to medium and cook until the skin is crispy, about 6-7 minutes.
4. Flip the duck breasts over and cook for an additional 2 minutes.
5. Transfer the skillet to the oven and roast for 5-7 minutes for medium-rare.
6. Remove the duck from the skillet and let rest.
7. In the same skillet, add cherries, red wine, balsamic vinegar, honey, and thyme. Bring to a simmer and cook until the sauce thickens.
8. Slice the duck and serve with the cherry sauce drizzled over the top.

Nutrition Info Per Serving (Serves 2):

- Calories: 460
- Fat: 22g
- Carbohydrates: 20g
- Protein: 40g
- Sodium: 220mg

Cooking Time:

- Preparation time: 10 minutes
- Cooking time: 20 minutes
- Total time: 30 minutes

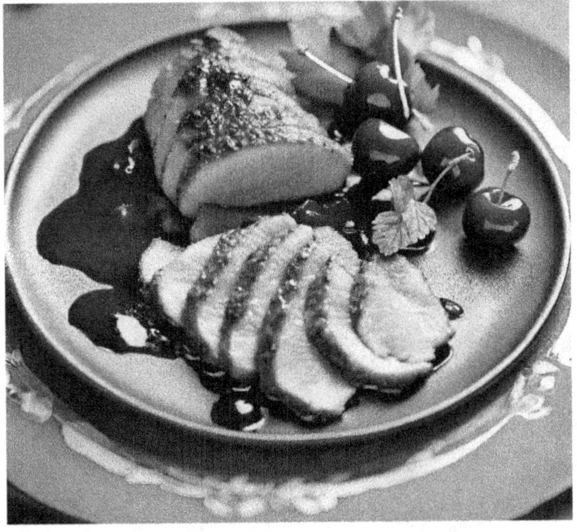

18. Turkey Meatball Soup
Ingredients:

- 1 lb ground turkey
- 1/2 cup breadcrumbs
- 1 egg
- 2 cloves garlic, minced
- 1/2 tsp salt
- 1/4 tsp pepper
- 1 tbsp olive oil
- 1 onion, chopped
- 2 carrots, diced
- 2 stalks celery, diced
- 6 cups chicken broth
- 1 tsp dried basil
- 1 tsp dried oregano

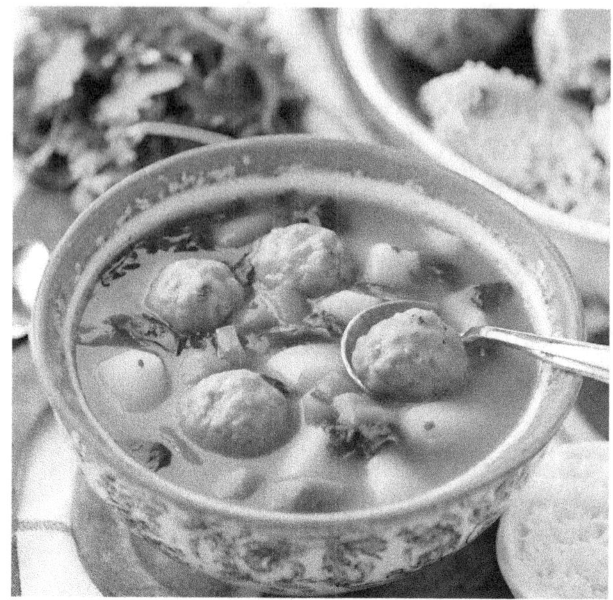

Instructions:

1. In a bowl, combine ground turkey, breadcrumbs, egg, garlic, salt, and pepper. Form into small meatballs.
2. Heat olive oil in a large pot over medium heat. Add meatballs and brown on all sides. Remove and set aside.
3. In the same pot, add onion, carrots, and celery. Cook until vegetables are softened, about 5 minutes.
4. Add chicken broth, basil, and oregano. Bring to a boil.
5. Return meatballs to the pot. Reduce heat and simmer for 20 minutes.
6. Serve hot.

Nutrition Info Per Serving (Serves 6):

- Calories: 220
- Fat: 10g
- Carbohydrates: 12g
- Protein: 20g
- Sodium: 950mg

Cooking Time:

- Preparation time: 15 minutes
- Cooking time: 30 minutes
- Total time: 45 minutes

19. Stuffed Chicken Breast with Spinach and Feta

Ingredients:

- 4 chicken breasts
- 1 cup spinach, cooked and squeezed dry
- 1/2 cup feta cheese, crumbled
- 2 cloves garlic, minced
- Salt and pepper to taste
- 2 tbsp olive oil

Instructions:

1. Preheat oven to 375°F (190°C).
2. Make a pocket in each chicken breast by slicing along one side.
3. Mix together spinach, feta, and garlic. Stuff this mixture into the pockets of the chicken breasts.
4. Season the outside of the chicken with salt and pepper.
5. Heat olive oil in a skillet over medium heat. Sear chicken on both sides until golden, about 3 minutes per side.
6. Transfer to the oven and bake for 20 minutes, or until the chicken is cooked through.
7. Serve hot.

Nutrition Info Per Serving (Serves 4):

- Calories: 330
- Fat: 18g
- Carbohydrates: 2g
- Protein: 38g
- Sodium: 450mg

Cooking Time:

- Preparation time: 10 minutes
- Cooking time: 30 minutes
- Total time: 40 minutes

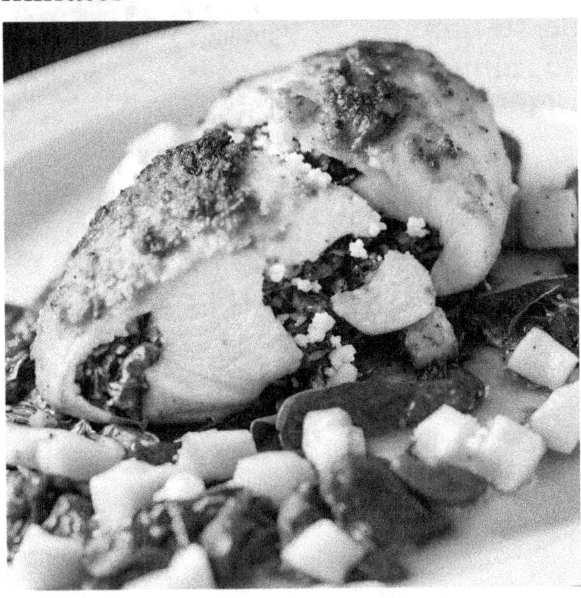

20. Grilled Skirt Steak with Chimichurri Sauce

Ingredients:

- 2 lbs skirt steak
- Salt and pepper to taste
- For the Chimichurri Sauce:
    - 1 cup fresh parsley, chopped
    - 1/4 cup fresh oregano, chopped
    - 3 cloves garlic, minced
    - 1/2 cup olive oil
    - 2 tbsp red wine vinegar
    - 1 tsp red pepper flakes
    - Salt to taste

Instructions:

1. Season the skirt steak with salt and pepper. Let it come to room temperature before grilling.
2. Preheat grill to high. Grill steak for 3-4 minutes per side for medium-rare.
3. Remove steak from grill and let rest for 5 minutes.
4. Meanwhile, combine all ingredients for the chimichurri sauce in a blender or food processor. Blend until smooth.
5. Slice the steak against the grain and serve with chimichurri sauce drizzled over the top.

Nutrition Info Per Serving (Serves 4):

- Calories: 580
- Fat: 44g
- Carbohydrates: 3g
- Protein: 42g
- Sodium: 120mg

Cooking Time:

- Preparation time: 10 minutes
- Cooking time: 10 minutes
- Total time: 20 minutes

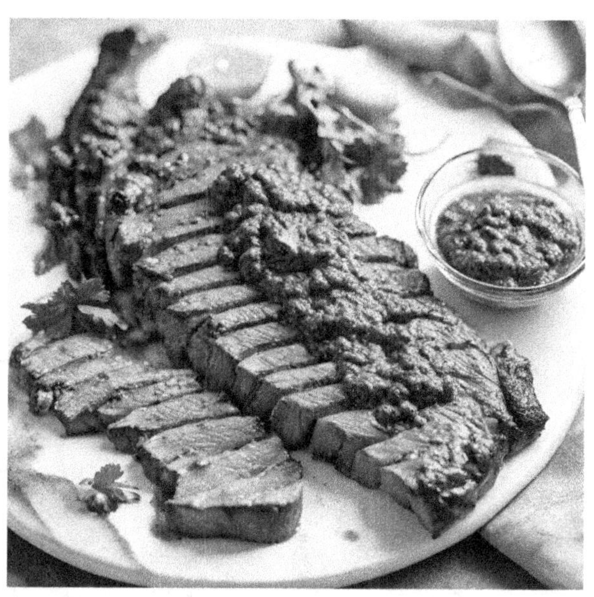

21. Italian Herb Chicken with Mediterranean Vegetables

Ingredients:

- 4 boneless, skinless chicken breasts
- 1 zucchini, sliced
- 1 red bell pepper, sliced
- 1 yellow bell pepper, sliced
- 1 red onion, sliced
- 2 tbsp olive oil
- 1 tsp dried oregano
- 1 tsp dried basil
- 1 tsp dried thyme
- Salt and pepper to taste
- Fresh basil for garnish

Instructions:

1. Preheat the oven to 375°F (190°C).
2. In a large baking dish, arrange the zucchini, bell peppers, and red onion. Drizzle with 1 tablespoon of olive oil and sprinkle with salt and pepper.
3. In a small bowl, combine the oregano, basil, thyme, salt, and pepper.
4. Rub the chicken breasts with the remaining olive oil and coat with the herb mixture.
5. Place the seasoned chicken breasts on top of the vegetables in the baking dish.
6. Bake in the preheated oven for 25-30 minutes, or until the chicken is fully cooked and the vegetables are tender.
7. Garnish with fresh basil before serving.

Nutrition Info Per Serving (Serves 4):

- Calories: 280
- Fat: 10g
- Carbohydrates: 8g
- Protein: 38g
- Sodium: 200mg

Cooking Time:

- Preparation time: 10 minutes
- Cooking time: 30 minutes
- Total time: 40 minutes

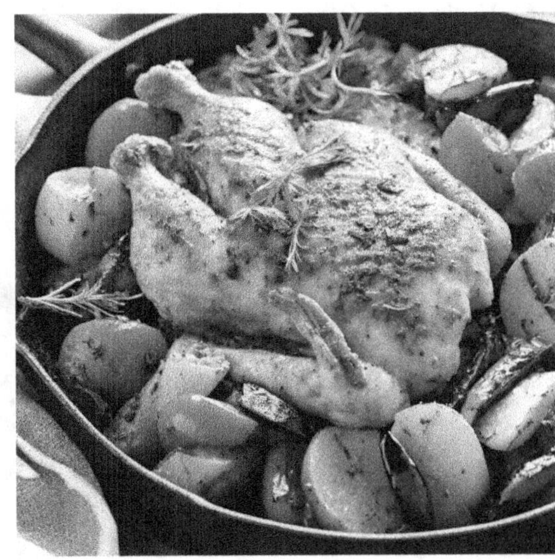

22. Braised Beef Short Ribs

Ingredients:

- 2 lbs beef short ribs
- 2 cups beef broth
- 1 cup red wine
- 1 onion, chopped
- 2 carrots, chopped
- 2 stalks celery, chopped
- 3 cloves garlic, minced
- 2 tbsp tomato paste
- 1 tbsp olive oil
- Salt and pepper to taste
- Fresh thyme and rosemary

Instructions:

1. Preheat the oven to 325°F (163°C).
2. Season the short ribs with salt and pepper.
3. Heat olive oil in a large oven-proof pot over medium-high heat. Brown the ribs on all sides, then remove and set aside.
4. In the same pot, add onion, carrots, celery, and garlic. Cook until softened.
5. Stir in tomato paste, and then add red wine and beef broth. Bring to a simmer.
6. Return the ribs to the pot, and add thyme and rosemary.
7. Cover and transfer to the oven. Braise for 2.5 to 3 hours, until the meat is very tender.
8. Serve the ribs with the braising liquid as a sauce.

Nutrition Info Per Serving (Serves 4):

- Calories: 560
- Fat: 42g
- Carbohydrates: 8g
- Protein: 32g
- Sodium: 450mg

Cooking Time:

- Preparation time: 20 minutes
- Cooking time: 3 hours
- Total time: 3 hours 20 minutes

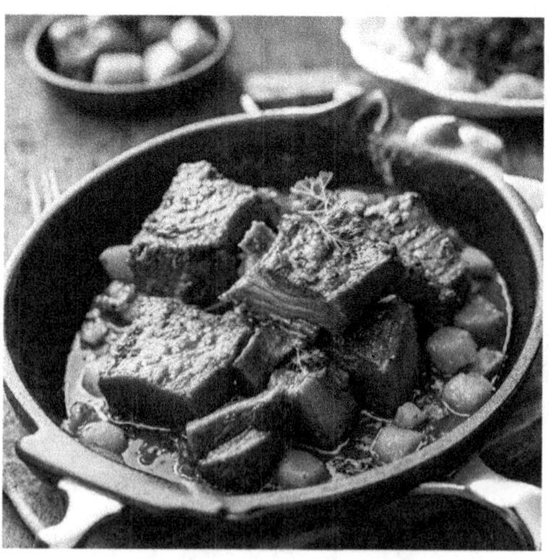

23. Venison Stew with Juniper Berries

Ingredients:

- 2 lbs venison, cubed
- 3 cups beef broth
- 1 cup red wine
- 1 onion, chopped
- 2 carrots, diced
- 2 potatoes, cubed
- 1/4 cup juniper berries
- 2 tbsp olive oil
- Salt and pepper to taste
- 2 bay leaves

Instructions:

1. Heat olive oil in a large pot over medium-high heat. Brown the venison cubes, then remove and set aside.
2. In the same pot, add onions and carrots, cooking until softened.
3. Return the venison to the pot along with potatoes, juniper berries, bay leaves, red wine, and beef broth.
4. Bring to a boil, then reduce heat to low and simmer covered for 2 hours, or until the meat is tender.
5. Season with salt and pepper to taste.
6. Serve hot.

Nutrition Info Per Serving (Serves 4):

- Calories: 450
- Fat: 10g
- Carbohydrates: 20g
- Protein: 50g
- Sodium: 450mg

Cooking Time:

- Preparation time: 15 minutes
- Cooking time: 2 hours
- Total time: 2 hours 15 minutes

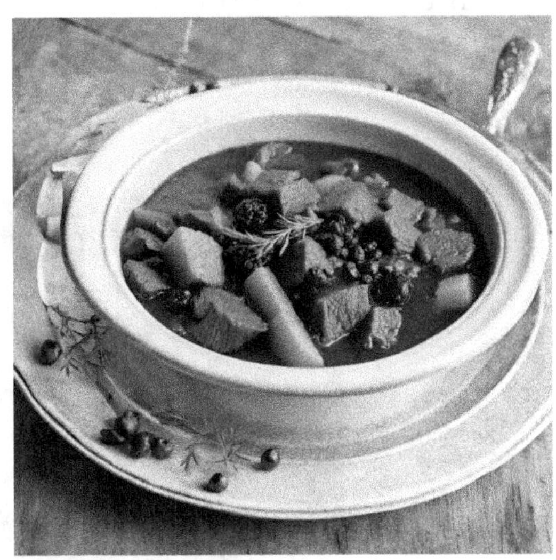

24. Beef Carpaccio with Arugula Salad

Ingredients:

- 1 lb beef tenderloin, thinly sliced
- 2 cups arugula
- 1/4 cup shaved Parmesan cheese
- 1/4 cup extra virgin olive oil
- 2 tbsp lemon juice
- Salt and pepper to taste
- Capers (optional)

Instructions:

1. Arrange the thinly sliced beef tenderloin on a serving plate.
2. In a bowl, whisk together olive oil, lemon juice, salt, and pepper.
3. Toss the arugula in the dressing and place on top of the beef.
4. Sprinkle shaved Parmesan and capers over the salad.
5. Serve immediately.

Nutrition Info Per Serving (Serves 4):

- Calories: 290
- Fat: 22g
- Carbohydrates: 2g
- Protein: 20g
- Sodium: 180mg

Cooking Time:

- Preparation time: 10 minutes
- Cooking time: 0 minutes
- Total time: 10 minutes

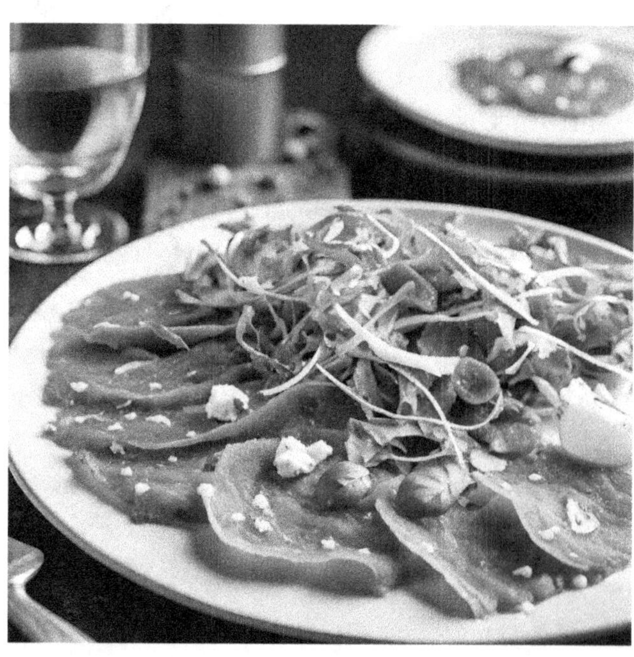

25. Chicken Pad Thai

Ingredients:

- 1 lb chicken breast, sliced
- 8 oz rice noodles
- 1/4 cup tamarind paste
- 2 tbsp fish sauce
- 1 tbsp soy sauce
- 2 tbsp brown sugar
- 2 cloves garlic, minced
- 1/4 cup peanuts, chopped
- 1 egg, beaten
- 1 cup bean sprouts
- 1/4 cup green onions, chopped
- 2 tbsp vegetable oil
- Lime wedges for serving

Instructions:

1. Soak rice noodles in warm water until soft, then drain.
2. In a small bowl, mix tamarind paste, fish sauce, soy sauce, and brown sugar.
3. Heat oil in a wok or large skillet over medium-high heat. Add garlic and chicken. Cook until chicken is done.
4. Push chicken to the side of the wok, and pour the beaten egg into the center. Scramble the egg until set.
5. Add noodles and sauce mixture. Toss everything together and cook for a few minutes until noodles are tender.
6. Stir in bean sprouts and green onions. Cook for another minute.
7. Serve hot, garnished with chopped peanuts and lime wedges.

Nutrition Info Per Serving (Serves 4):

- Calories: 520
- Fat: 18g
- Carbohydrates: 62g
- Protein: 32g
- Sodium: 1100mg

Cooking Time:

- Preparation time: 20 minutes
- Cooking time: 15 minutes
- Total time: 35 minutes

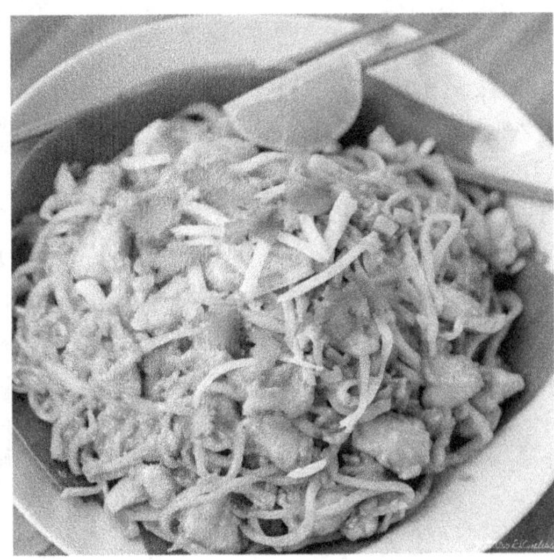

Vegetables

1. Spaghetti Squash with Tomato Sauce and Olives
Ingredients:
- 1 spaghetti squash, halved lengthwise and seeds removed
- 1 cup tomato sauce
- 1/2 cup black olives, sliced
- 2 cloves garlic, minced
- 1 tbsp olive oil
- Salt and pepper to taste
- Fresh basil for garnish

Instructions:
1. Preheat the oven to 400°F (200°C).
2. Brush the cut sides of the spaghetti squash with olive oil and season with salt and pepper. Place cut-side down on a baking sheet.
3. Roast in the preheated oven for 40 minutes, or until tender.
4. While the squash is roasting, heat the tomato sauce with garlic and olives in a saucepan over medium heat.
5. Once the squash is done, use a fork to scrape out the strands into a bowl.
6. Top the spaghetti squash with the warm tomato sauce and olives.
7. Garnish with fresh basil and serve.

Nutrition Info Per Serving (Serves 4):
- Calories: 140
- Fat: 7g
- Carbohydrates: 20g
- Protein: 3g
- Sodium: 400mg

Cooking Time:
- Preparation time: 10 minutes
- Cooking time: 40 minutes
- Total time: 50 minutes

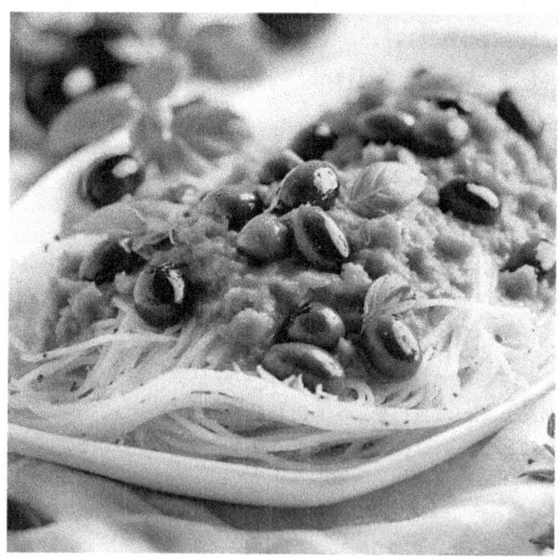

2. Japanese-style Steamed Vegetables with Miso Dressing

Ingredients:

- 2 cups broccoli florets
- 2 carrots, sliced into matchsticks
- 1 bell pepper, sliced
- 1/4 cup miso paste
- 2 tbsp rice vinegar
- 1 tbsp soy sauce
- 1 tbsp honey
- 1 tsp sesame oil
- 1 tbsp water
- Sesame seeds for garnish

Instructions:

1. Steam the broccoli, carrots, and bell pepper until just tender, about 5-7 minutes.
2. In a small bowl, whisk together miso paste, rice vinegar, soy sauce, honey, sesame oil, and water until smooth.
3. Drizzle the miso dressing over the steamed vegetables.
4. Garnish with sesame seeds and serve immediately.

Nutrition Info Per Serving (Serves 4):

- Calories: 120
- Fat: 3g
- Carbohydrates: 20g
- Protein: 5g
- Sodium: 630mg

Cooking Time:

- Preparation time: 10 minutes
- Cooking time: 7 minutes
- Total time: 17 minutes

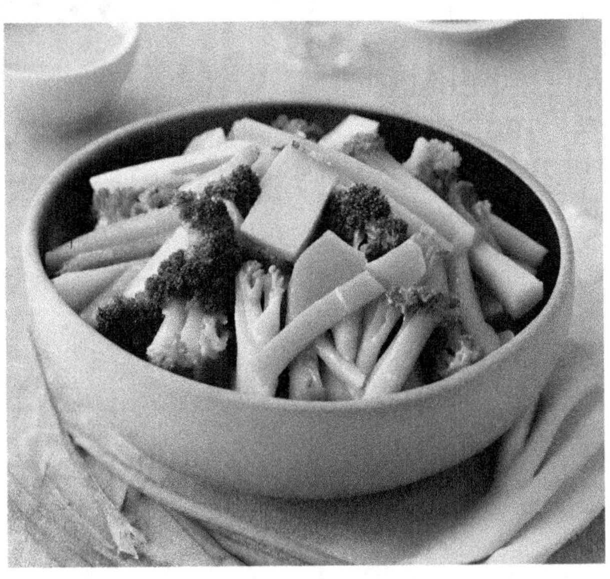

3. Curried Vegetable and Chickpea Stew

Ingredients:

- 1 onion, chopped
- 2 cloves garlic, minced
- 1 tbsp ginger, minced
- 2 tbsp curry powder
- 1 can (15 oz) chickpeas, drained and rinsed
- 1 can (14.5 oz) diced tomatoes
- 1 cup coconut milk
- 2 potatoes, cubed
- 2 carrots, sliced
- 1 bell pepper, chopped
- 2 cups spinach leaves
- 2 tbsp olive oil
- Salt to taste

Instructions:

1. Heat olive oil in a large pot over medium heat. Add onion, garlic, and ginger, sautéing until onion is translucent.
2. Stir in curry powder and cook for another minute.
3. Add chickpeas, diced tomatoes, coconut milk, potatoes, carrots, and bell pepper. Bring to a boil, then reduce heat and simmer for 20 minutes, or until vegetables are tender.
4. Stir in spinach and cook until wilted.
5. Season with salt to taste and serve.

Nutrition Info Per Serving (Serves 6):

- Calories: 250
- Fat: 10g
- Carbohydrates: 35g
- Protein: 8g
- Sodium: 300mg

Cooking Time:

- Preparation time: 15 minutes
- Cooking time: 25 minutes
- Total time: 40 minutes

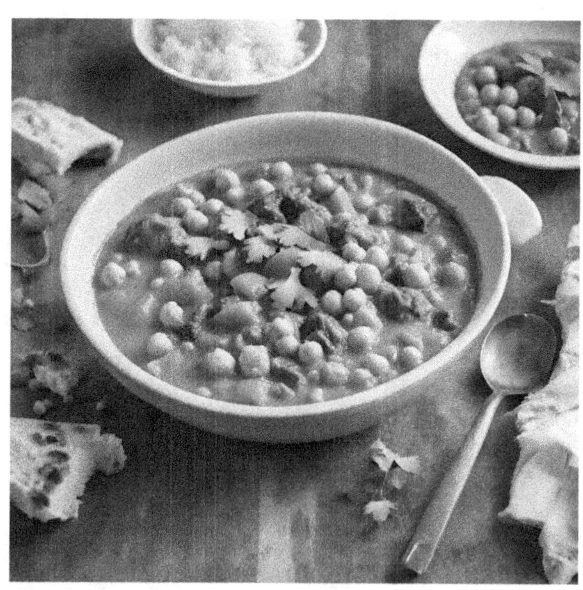

4. Pan-Seared Brussels Sprouts with Pomegranate Seeds

Ingredients:

- 1 lb Brussels sprouts, halved
- 1 tbsp olive oil
- Salt and pepper to taste
- 1/2 cup pomegranate seeds

Instructions:

1. Heat olive oil in a large skillet over medium-high heat.
2. Add Brussels sprouts, cut side down, and cook without stirring for about 5 minutes until the cut sides are golden brown.
3. Stir and continue cooking for another 5-7 minutes until tender.
4. Season with salt and pepper.
5. Remove from heat and sprinkle with pomegranate seeds.
6. Serve immediately.

Nutrition Info Per Serving (Serves 4):

- Calories: 120
- Fat: 4g
- Carbohydrates: 18g
- Protein: 5g
- Sodium: 30mg

Cooking Time:

- Preparation time: 5 minutes
- Cooking time: 12 minutes
- Total time: 17 minutes

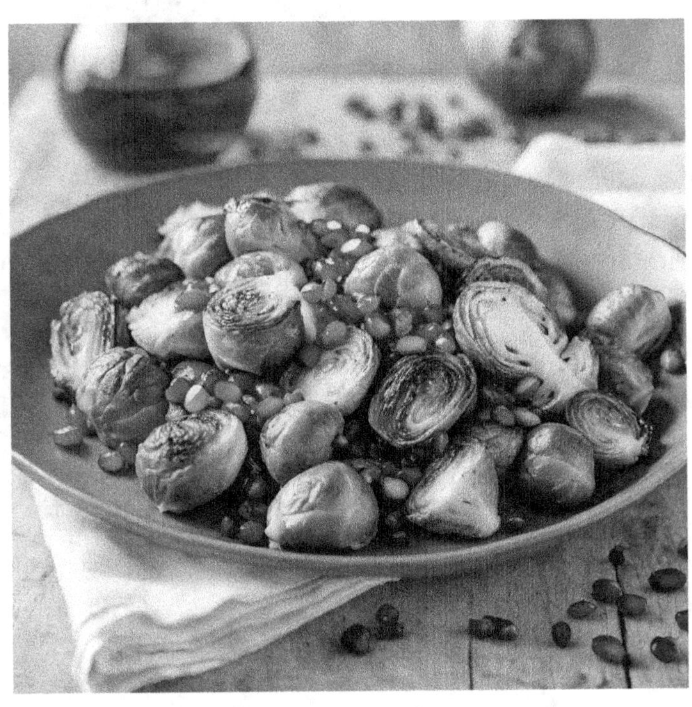

5. Stuffed Acorn Squash with Wild Rice and Cranberries

Ingredients:

- 2 acorn squash, halved and seeds removed
- 1 cup wild rice, cooked
- 1/2 cup dried cranberries
- 1/4 cup pecans, chopped
- 1 onion, diced
- 1 celery stalk, diced
- 2 tbsp olive oil
- Salt and pepper to taste
- Fresh thyme for garnish

Instructions:

1. Preheat the oven to 375°F (190°C).
2. Brush the inside of the acorn squash halves with 1 tbsp olive oil and season with salt and pepper. Place cut-side down on a baking sheet.
3. Roast in the preheated oven for 25 minutes, or until tender.
4. Meanwhile, heat the remaining olive oil in a skillet. Add onion and celery, and sauté until soft.
5. Mix the sautéed vegetables with cooked wild rice, cranberries, and pecans.
6. Turn the roasted squash halves cut-side up and stuff with the rice mixture.
7. Return to the oven and bake for another 10 minutes.
8. Garnish with fresh thyme and serve.

Nutrition Info Per Serving (Serves 4):

- Calories: 300
- Fat: 10g
- Carbohydrates: 50g
- Protein: 5g
- Sodium: 150mg

Cooking Time:

- Preparation time: 15 minutes
- Cooking time: 35 minutes
- Total time: 50 minutes

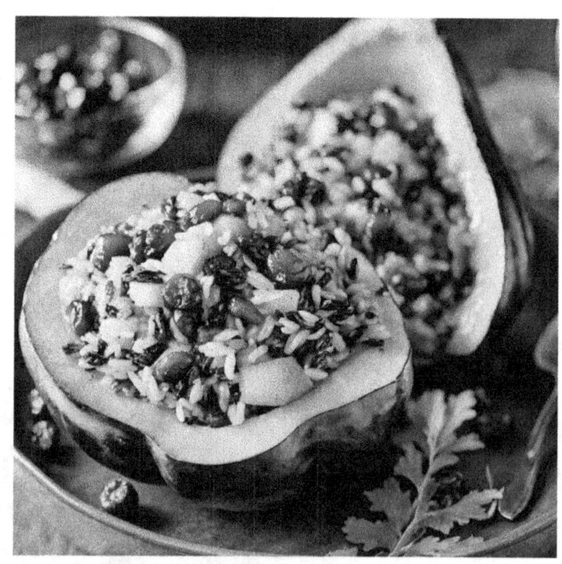

6. Garlic Braised Greens (Collards, Mustard, or Swiss Chard)

Ingredients:

- 1 lb greens (collard greens, mustard greens, or Swiss chard), stems removed and leaves chopped
- 3 cloves garlic, minced
- 2 tbsp olive oil
- 1/2 cup vegetable broth
- Salt and pepper to taste
- 1 tbsp apple cider vinegar

Instructions:

1. Heat olive oil in a large pot over medium heat. Add garlic and sauté until fragrant, about 1 minute.
2. Add the chopped greens and stir to coat with oil and garlic.
3. Pour in vegetable broth, cover, and reduce heat to low. Simmer for about 25-30 minutes for collard or mustard greens, or 15 minutes for Swiss chard, until the greens are tender.
4. Season with salt, pepper, and apple cider vinegar.
5. Serve warm.

Nutrition Info Per Serving (Serves 4):

- Calories: 90
- Fat: 7g
- Carbohydrates: 6g
- Protein: 3g
- Sodium: 200mg

Cooking Time:

- Preparation time: 10 minutes
- Cooking time: 30 minutes
- Total time: 40 minutes

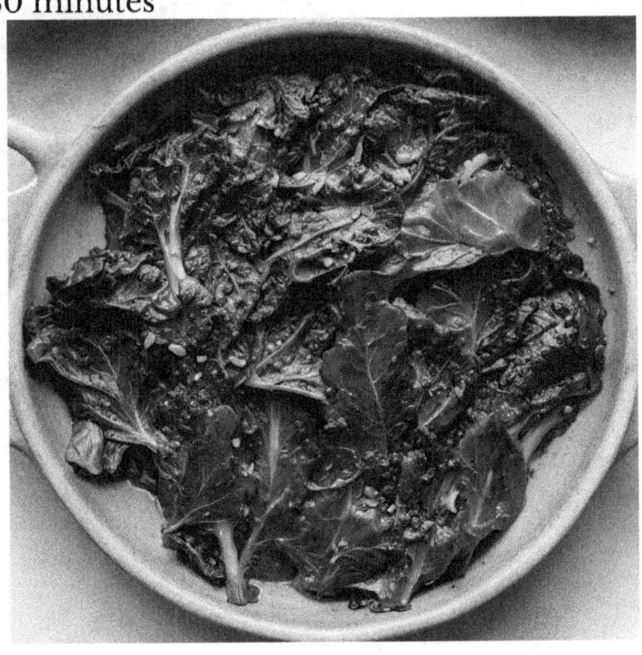

7. Sweet Potato and Black Bean Chili

Ingredients:

- 2 large sweet potatoes, peeled and cubed
- 1 can (15 oz) black beans, drained and rinsed
- 1 onion, chopped
- 2 cloves garlic, minced
- 1 bell pepper, chopped
- 1 can (14.5 oz) diced tomatoes
- 2 tbsp chili powder
- 1 tsp cumin
- 1/2 tsp paprika
- 3 cups vegetable broth
- 2 tbsp olive oil
- Salt and pepper to taste
- Fresh cilantro for garnish

Instructions:

1. Heat olive oil in a large pot over medium heat. Add onion, garlic, and bell pepper, sautéing until softened.
2. Stir in spices and cook for another minute until fragrant.
3. Add sweet potatoes, black beans, diced tomatoes, and vegetable broth. Bring to a boil.
4. Reduce heat to simmer and cook uncovered for about 25 minutes, or until the sweet potatoes are tender.
5. Season with salt and pepper. Garnish with fresh cilantro before serving.

Nutrition Info Per Serving (Serves 6):

- Calories: 230
- Fat: 5g
- Carbohydrates: 40g
- Protein: 8g
- Sodium: 400mg

Cooking Time:

- Preparation time: 10 minutes
- Cooking time: 30 minutes
- Total time: 40 minutes

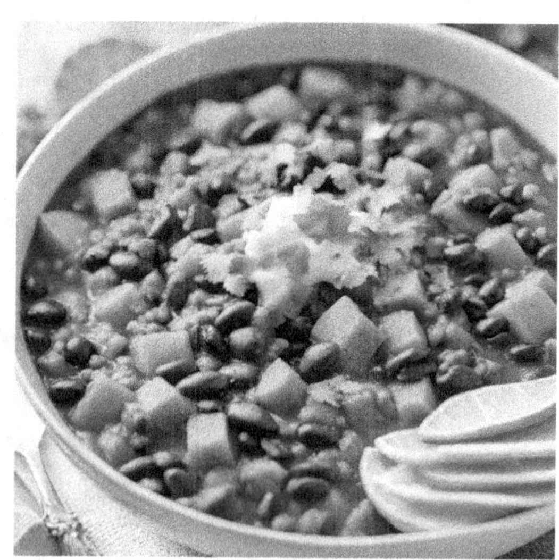

8. Fennel and Citrus Salad

Ingredients:

- 1 fennel bulb, thinly sliced
- 2 oranges, peeled and segments cut out
- 1 grapefruit, peeled and segments cut out
- 1/4 red onion, thinly sliced
- 2 tbsp olive oil
- 2 tbsp lemon juice
- Salt and pepper to taste
- Fresh mint leaves, for garnish

Instructions:

1. In a salad bowl, combine sliced fennel, orange segments, grapefruit segments, and red onion.
2. In a small bowl, whisk together olive oil and lemon juice. Season with salt and pepper.
3. Drizzle the dressing over the salad and gently toss to coat.
4. Garnish with fresh mint leaves.
5. Serve chilled or at room temperature.

Nutrition Info Per Serving (Serves 4):

- Calories: 140
- Fat: 7g
- Carbohydrates: 20g
- Protein: 2g
- Sodium: 75mg

Cooking Time:

- Preparation time: 15 minutes
- Total time: 15 minutes

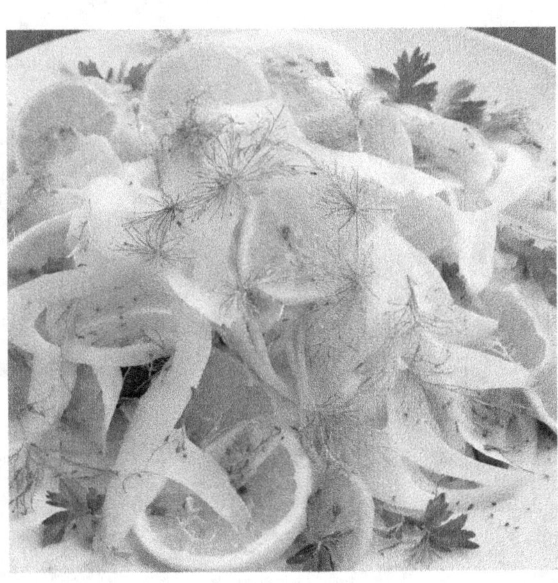

9. Balsamic Glazed Beets

Ingredients:

- 4 medium beets, peeled and cubed
- 2 tbsp olive oil
- 2 tbsp balsamic vinegar
- 1 tbsp honey
- Salt and pepper to taste
- Fresh parsley, chopped for garnish

Instructions:

1. Preheat the oven to 400°F (200°C).
2. Toss the beets with olive oil, salt, and pepper. Spread on a baking sheet and roast for about 30 minutes, or until tender.
3. In a small saucepan, heat balsamic vinegar and honey over medium heat. Simmer until reduced by half and thickened, about 5 minutes.
4. Drizzle the balsamic glaze over the roasted beets.
5. Garnish with chopped parsley.
6. Serve warm or at room temperature.

Nutrition Info Per Serving (Serves 4):

- Calories: 150
- Fat: 7g
- Carbohydrates: 20g
- Protein: 2g
- Sodium: 110mg

Cooking Time:

- Preparation time: 10 minutes
- Cooking time: 35 minutes
- Total time: 45 minutes

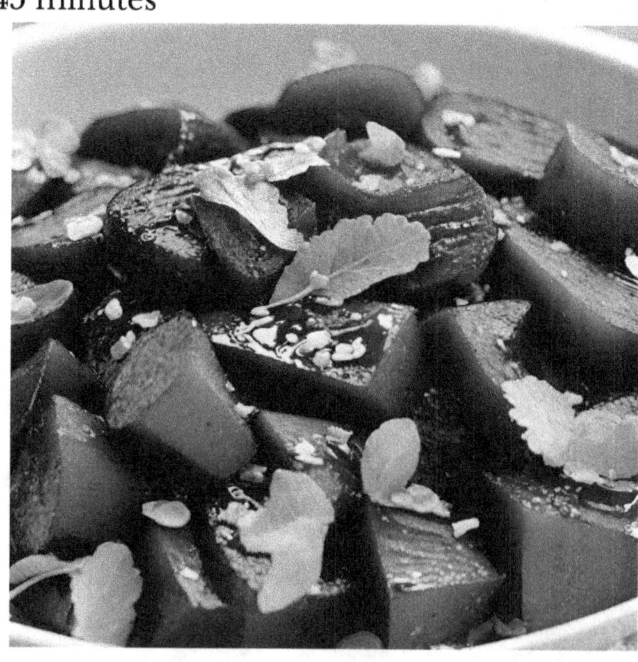

10. Roasted Garlic Cauliflower

Ingredients:

- 1 head cauliflower, cut into florets
- 3 tbsp olive oil
- 3 cloves garlic, minced
- Salt and pepper to taste
- Fresh parsley, chopped for garnish

Instructions:

1. Preheat the oven to 425°F (220°C).
2. In a large bowl, toss the cauliflower florets with olive oil, minced garlic, salt, and pepper.
3. Spread the cauliflower on a baking sheet in a single layer.
4. Roast in the preheated oven for 25-30 minutes, stirring halfway through, until golden and tender.
5. Garnish with chopped parsley before serving.

Nutrition Info Per Serving (Serves 4):

- Calories: 120
- Fat: 10g
- Carbohydrates: 8g
- Protein: 3g
- Sodium: 75mg

Cooking Time:

- Preparation time: 10 minutes
- Cooking time: 30 minutes
- Total time: 40 minutes

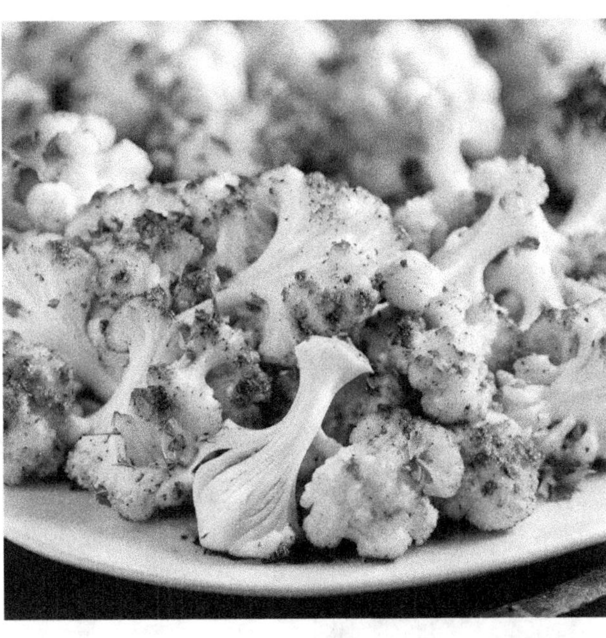

11. Spiced Lentil Stew with Carrots

Ingredients:

- 1 cup dried lentils, rinsed
- 4 cups vegetable broth
- 2 carrots, diced
- 1 onion, chopped
- 2 cloves garlic, minced
- 1 tsp cumin
- 1 tsp coriander
- 1/2 tsp smoked paprika
- 2 tbsp olive oil
- Salt and pepper to taste
- Fresh cilantro, chopped for garnish

Instructions:

1. Heat olive oil in a large pot over medium heat. Add onion and garlic, sauté until translucent.
2. Stir in carrots and spices, cooking for another 2 minutes.
3. Add lentils and vegetable broth. Bring to a boil, then reduce heat to low and simmer for 25-30 minutes, until lentils are tender.
4. Season with salt and pepper.
5. Garnish with chopped cilantro before serving.

Nutrition Info Per Serving (Serves 4):

- Calories: 240
- Fat: 7g
- Carbohydrates: 33g
- Protein: 13g
- Sodium: 480mg

Cooking Time:

- Preparation time: 10 minutes
- Cooking time: 30 minutes
- Total time: 40 minutes

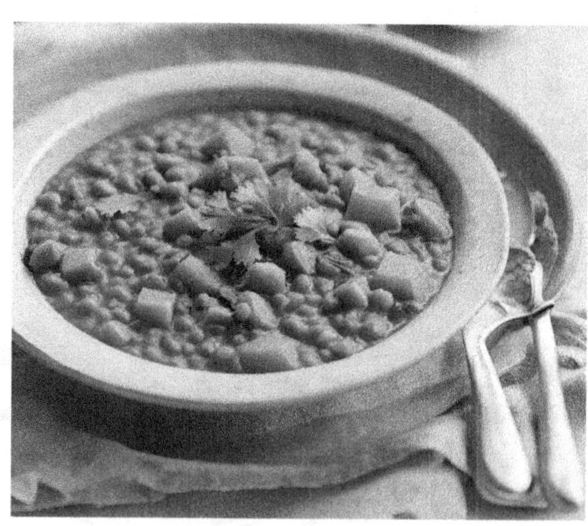

12. Red Cabbage Slaw with Apple Cider Vinaigrette

Ingredients:

- 1/2 head red cabbage, shredded
- 1 carrot, grated
- 1 apple, thinly sliced
- 1/4 cup apple cider vinegar
- 2 tbsp olive oil
- 1 tbsp honey
- Salt and pepper to taste

Instructions:

1. In a large bowl, combine the shredded cabbage, grated carrot, and sliced apple.
2. In a small bowl, whisk together apple cider vinegar, olive oil, honey, salt, and pepper to make the dressing.
3. Pour the dressing over the cabbage mixture and toss well to coat.
4. Refrigerate for at least 30 minutes before serving to allow flavors to meld.

Nutrition Info Per Serving (Serves 4):

- Calories: 140
- Fat: 7g
- Carbohydrates: 20g
- Protein: 2g
- Sodium: 50mg

Cooking Time:

- Preparation time: 10 minutes
- Resting time: 30 minutes
- Total time: 40 minutes

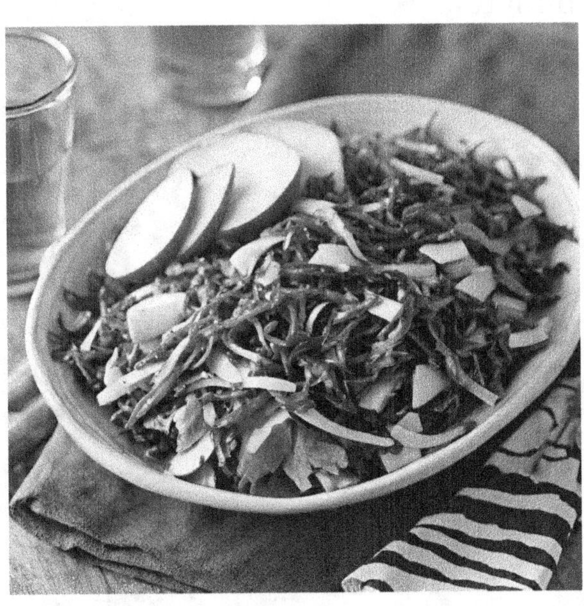

13. Creamy Avocado Pasta

Ingredients:

- 2 ripe avocados, peeled and pitted
- 2 cloves garlic, minced
- Juice of 1 lemon
- 1/4 cup olive oil
- Salt and pepper to taste
- 12 oz spaghetti or your choice of pasta
- Fresh basil, chopped for garnish
- Grated Parmesan cheese (optional)

Instructions:

1. Cook the pasta according to package instructions until al dente. Drain and set aside.
2. In a blender, combine avocados, garlic, lemon juice, olive oil, salt, and pepper. Blend until smooth.
3. Toss the pasta with the avocado sauce until evenly coated.
4. Garnish with chopped basil and grated Parmesan cheese if desired.
5. Serve immediately.

Nutrition Info Per Serving (Serves 4):

- Calories: 550
- Fat: 30g
- Carbohydrates: 60g
- Protein: 12g
- Sodium: 25mg

Cooking Time:

- Preparation time: 10 minutes
- Cooking time: 10 minutes
- Total time: 20 minutes

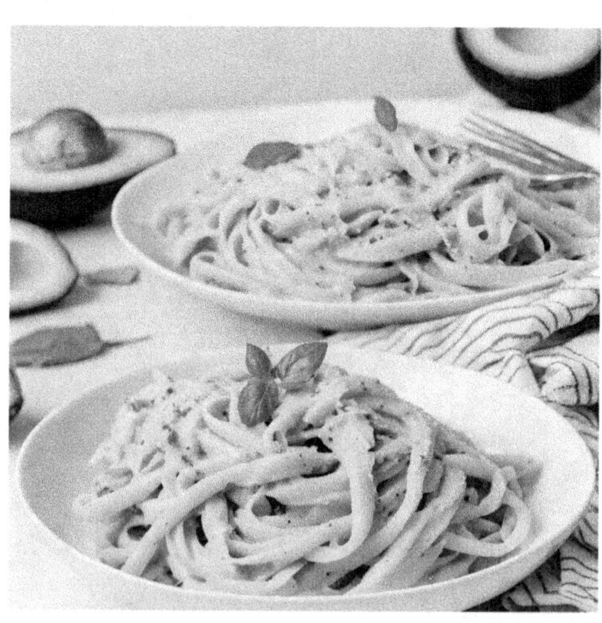

14. Grilled Corn on the Cob with Chili Lime Butter
Ingredients:
- 4 ears of corn, husks removed
- 4 tbsp butter, softened
- 1 lime, zested and juiced
- 1/2 tsp chili powder
- Salt to taste
- Fresh cilantro, chopped for garnish

Instructions:
1. Preheat your grill to medium-high heat.
2. In a small bowl, combine butter, lime zest, lime juice, chili powder, and salt. Mix well to create chili lime butter.
3. Brush each ear of corn generously with the chili lime butter.
4. Place corn on the grill and cook, turning occasionally, until the kernels are tender and charred in spots, about 10-12 minutes.
5. Remove from the grill and sprinkle with fresh cilantro before serving.

Nutrition Info Per Serving (Serves 4):
- Calories: 180
- Fat: 11g
- Carbohydrates: 21g
- Protein: 3g
- Sodium: 85mg

Cooking Time:
- Preparation time: 5 minutes
- Cooking time: 12 minutes
- Total time: 17 minutes

15. Vegetable Stir Fry with Tamari Sauce

Ingredients:

- 2 cups broccoli florets
- 1 red bell pepper, sliced
- 1 yellow bell pepper, sliced
- 1 carrot, sliced thinly
- 1 zucchini, sliced
- 2 tbsp olive oil
- 1/4 cup tamari sauce
- 2 cloves garlic, minced
- 1 tbsp ginger, minced
- 1 tbsp sesame seeds

Instructions:

1. Heat olive oil in a large skillet or wok over medium-high heat.
2. Add garlic and ginger, and sauté for about 30 seconds until fragrant.
3. Add all the vegetables to the skillet. Stir fry for about 5-7 minutes until just tender but still crisp.
4. Pour tamari sauce over the vegetables and stir to combine. Cook for an additional 2 minutes.
5. Sprinkle sesame seeds over the stir fry before serving.

Nutrition Info Per Serving (Serves 4):

- Calories: 160
- Fat: 8g
- Carbohydrates: 18g
- Protein: 6g
- Sodium: 800mg

Cooking Time:

- Preparation time: 10 minutes
- Cooking time: 10 minutes
- Total time: 20 minutes

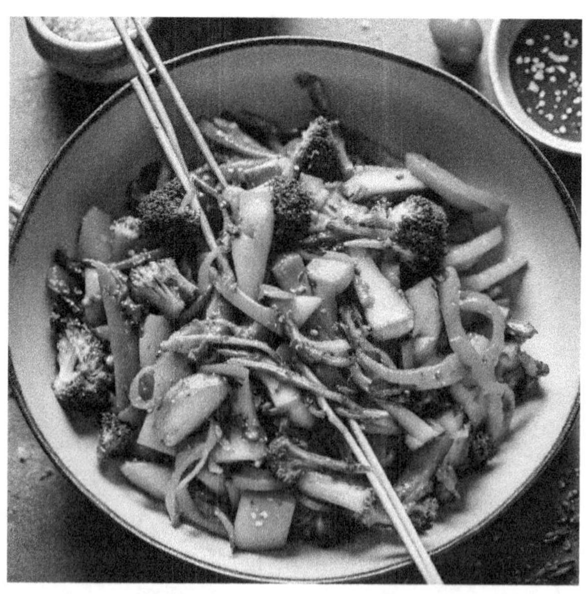

16. Tomato Gazpacho

Ingredients:

- 6 ripe tomatoes, chopped
- 1 cucumber, peeled and chopped
- 1 bell pepper, chopped
- 1 onion, chopped
- 2 cloves garlic, minced
- 3 cups tomato juice
- 1/4 cup red wine vinegar
- 1/4 cup olive oil
- Salt and pepper to taste
- Fresh basil, chopped for garnish

Instructions:

1. In a blender, combine tomatoes, cucumber, bell pepper, onion, garlic, and half the tomato juice. Blend until smooth.
2. Pour the blended mixture into a large bowl. Stir in the remaining tomato juice, red wine vinegar, and olive oil. Season with salt and pepper.
3. Chill in the refrigerator for at least 2 hours before serving.
4. Garnish with fresh basil when serving.

Nutrition Info Per Serving (Serves 6):

- Calories: 140
- Fat: 9g
- Carbohydrates: 15g
- Protein: 3g
- Sodium: 30mg

Cooking Time:

- Preparation time: 15 minutes
- Chilling time: 2 hours
- Total time: 2 hours 15 minutes

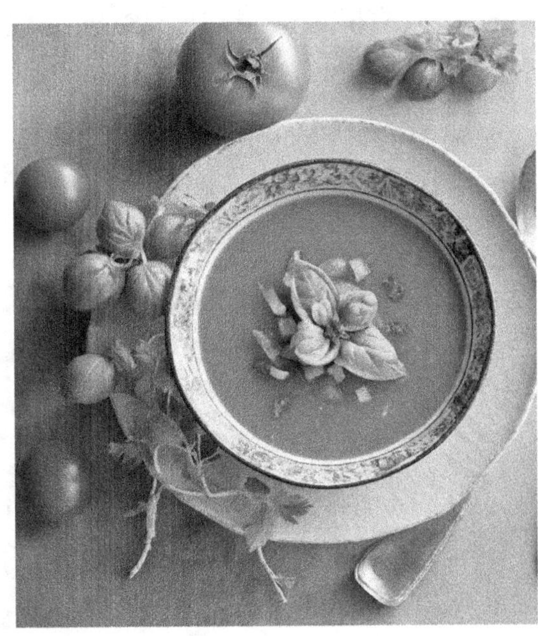

17. Spinach and Goat Cheese Tart

Ingredients:

- 1 pre-made pie crust
- 10 oz spinach, washed and chopped
- 1 onion, thinly sliced
- 2 cloves garlic, minced
- 4 oz goat cheese, crumbled
- 3 eggs, beaten
- 1 cup milk
- 2 tbsp olive oil
- Salt and pepper to taste
- Nutmeg, a pinch

Instructions:

1. Preheat the oven to 375°F (190°C).
2. In a skillet, heat olive oil over medium heat. Add onion and garlic, sauté until soft. Add spinach and cook until wilted. Remove from heat.
3. Spread the spinach mixture evenly over the pie crust. Sprinkle goat cheese on top.
4. In a bowl, whisk together eggs, milk, salt, pepper, and nutmeg. Pour this mixture over the spinach and cheese.
5. Bake in the preheated oven for 35-40 minutes, or until the custard is set and the top is lightly golden.
6. Let cool for a few minutes before slicing and serving.

Nutrition Info Per Serving (Serves 6):

- Calories: 320
- Fat: 21g
- Carbohydrates: 22g
- Protein: 12g
- Sodium: 400mg

Cooking Time:

- Preparation time: 15 minutes
- Cooking time: 40 minutes
- Total time: 55 minutes

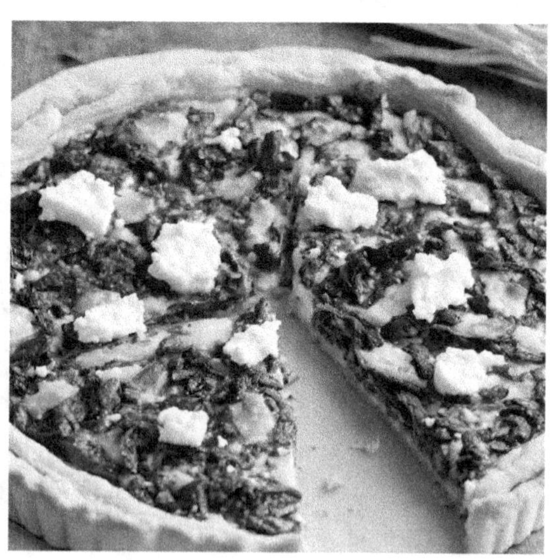

18. Sautéed Green Beans with Garlic and Almonds

Ingredients:

- 1 lb green beans, trimmed
- 3 tbsp olive oil
- 2 cloves garlic, minced
- 1/2 cup sliced almonds
- Salt and pepper to taste

Instructions:

1. Heat olive oil in a large skillet over medium heat.
2. Add the green beans and sauté for about 5 minutes, until they start to soften.
3. Add the minced garlic and sliced almonds, and continue to cook for another 5 minutes, or until the beans are tender and the almonds are lightly toasted.
4. Season with salt and pepper to taste.
5. Serve hot.

Nutrition Info Per Serving (Serves 4):

- Calories: 180
- Fat: 14g
- Carbohydrates: 10g
- Protein: 5g
- Sodium: 10mg

Cooking Time:

- Preparation time: 5 minutes
- Cooking time: 10 minutes
- Total time: 15 minutes

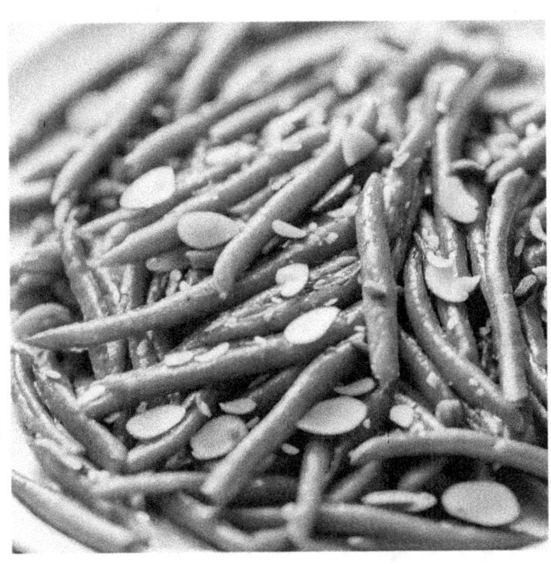

19. Mushroom Risotto with Parsley

Ingredients:

- 1 cup arborio rice
- 1 lb mushrooms, sliced
- 1 onion, finely chopped
- 2 cloves garlic, minced
- 4 cups vegetable broth
- 1/2 cup white wine
- 1/4 cup grated Parmesan cheese
- 2 tbsp olive oil
- 1/4 cup chopped parsley
- Salt and pepper to taste

Instructions:

1. In a saucepan, heat the vegetable broth over low heat.
2. In another saucepan, heat olive oil over medium heat. Add onion and garlic, and sauté until translucent.
3. Add the mushrooms and cook until they release their juices and begin to brown.
4. Stir in the rice and cook for 2 minutes until slightly toasted.
5. Add the white wine and cook until the liquid is mostly absorbed.
6. Begin adding the warm broth one cup at a time, stirring constantly, until each addition is absorbed before adding the next.
7. Once all the broth is used and the rice is creamy and al dente, stir in the Parmesan cheese, parsley, salt, and pepper.
8. Serve hot.

Nutrition Info Per Serving (Serves 4):

- Calories: 350
- Fat: 12g
- Carbohydrates: 50g
- Protein: 10g
- Sodium: 400mg

Cooking Time:

- Preparation time: 10 minutes
- Cooking time: 30 minutes
- Total time: 40 minutes

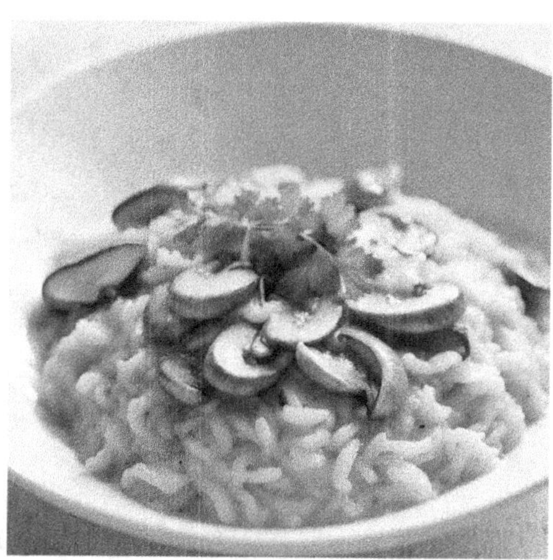

20. Spicy Stir-Fried Tofu with Broccoli

Ingredients:

- 1 lb firm tofu, drained and cubed
- 4 cups broccoli florets
- 2 tbsp sesame oil
- 2 cloves garlic, minced
- 2 tbsp soy sauce
- 1 tbsp chili sauce
- 1 tsp cornstarch mixed with 2 tbsp water
- Salt and pepper to taste

Instructions:

1. Heat sesame oil in a large skillet or wok over medium-high heat.
2. Add garlic and sauté for 30 seconds.
3. Add tofu and fry until golden on all sides.
4. Add broccoli and stir-fry for about 5 minutes, or until tender-crisp.
5. In a small bowl, mix soy sauce, chili sauce, and cornstarch mixture. Pour over the tofu and broccoli.
6. Cook for another 2 minutes, stirring constantly, until the sauce thickens and everything is evenly coated.
7. Season with salt and pepper to taste.
8. Serve hot.

Nutrition Info Per Serving (Serves 4):

- Calories: 220
- Fat: 12g
- Carbohydrates: 15g
- Protein: 15g
- Sodium: 630mg

Cooking Time:

- Preparation time: 10 minutes
- Cooking time: 10 minutes
- Total time: 20 minutes

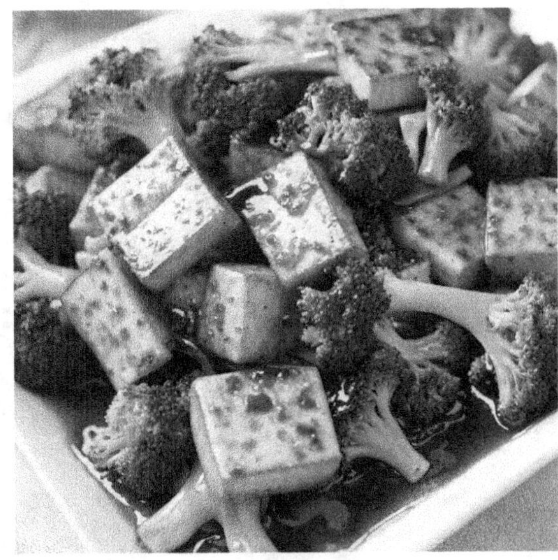

21. Kale Salad with Avocado and Pumpkin Seeds

Ingredients:

- 4 cups chopped kale, stems removed
- 1 ripe avocado, diced
- 1/4 cup pumpkin seeds
- 1 lemon, juiced
- 2 tbsp olive oil
- Salt and pepper to taste

Instructions:

1. In a large salad bowl, combine kale, avocado, and pumpkin seeds.
2. In a small bowl, whisk together lemon juice, olive oil, salt, and pepper.
3. Drizzle the dressing over the salad and toss well to coat.
4. Let the salad sit for about 10 minutes before serving to allow the kale to soften slightly.
5. Serve chilled or at room temperature.

Nutrition Info Per Serving (Serves 4):

- Calories: 200
- Fat: 15g
- Carbohydrates: 15g
- Protein: 6g
- Sodium: 50mg

Cooking Time:

- Preparation time: 10 minutes
- Total time: 10 minutes

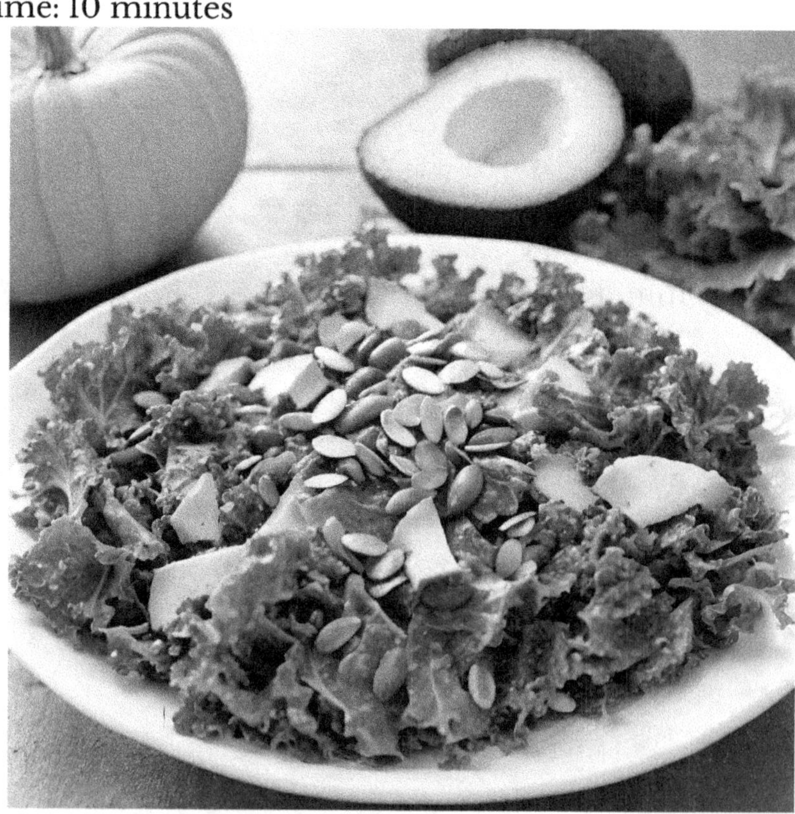

22. Eggplant Parmesan Stacks

Ingredients:

- 2 large eggplants, sliced into 1/2-inch rounds
- 1 cup marinara sauce
- 1 cup shredded mozzarella cheese
- 1/2 cup grated Parmesan cheese
- 1/4 cup fresh basil leaves, chopped
- 1/2 cup flour
- 2 eggs, beaten
- 1 cup breadcrumbs
- Salt and pepper to taste
- Olive oil for frying

Instructions:

1. Season eggplant slices with salt and let sit for 20 minutes to draw out moisture. Pat dry with paper towels.
2. Dredge each slice first in flour, then dip in beaten eggs, and finally coat with breadcrumbs.
3. Heat olive oil in a large skillet over medium heat. Fry the eggplant slices until golden on each side, about 2-3 minutes per side. Drain on paper towels.
4. Preheat the oven to 375°F (190°C).
5. On a baking sheet, place a slice of eggplant, top with a spoonful of marinara sauce, a sprinkle of mozzarella, and a little Parmesan. Repeat the layering with another slice of eggplant and more cheese.
6. Bake in the oven for 10-15 minutes, until the cheese is melted and bubbly.
7. Garnish with chopped basil before serving.

Nutrition Info Per Serving (Serves 6):

- Calories: 300
- Fat: 15g
- Carbohydrates: 30g
- Protein: 15g
- Sodium: 450mg

Cooking Time:

- Preparation time: 30 minutes
- Cooking time: 20 minutes
- Total time: 50 minutes

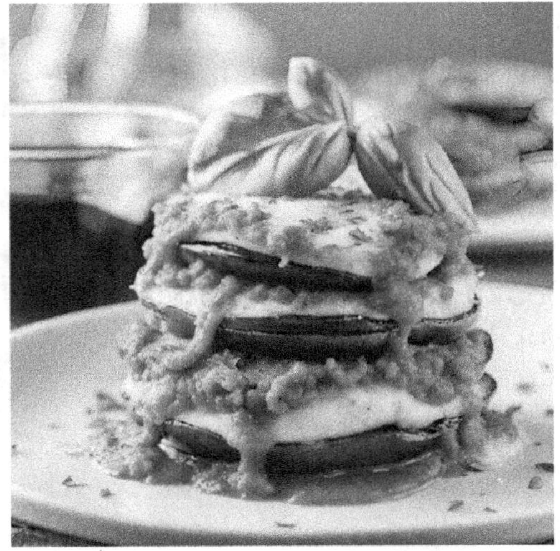

23. Stuffed Bell Peppers with Quinoa and Black Beans

Ingredients:

- 4 large bell peppers, tops cut off and seeds removed
- 1 cup cooked quinoa
- 1 can (15 oz) black beans, drained and rinsed
- 1 cup corn kernels
- 1 onion, chopped
- 2 cloves garlic, minced
- 1 cup tomato sauce
- 1 tsp chili powder
- 1 tsp cumin
- 1/2 cup shredded cheddar cheese
- 2 tbsp olive oil
- Salt and pepper to taste

Instructions:

1. Preheat the oven to 350°F (175°C).
2. Heat olive oil in a skillet over medium heat. Add onion and garlic, and sauté until softened.
3. Stir in quinoa, black beans, corn, tomato sauce, chili powder, and cumin. Cook until heated through.
4. Season the mixture with salt and pepper.
5. Stuff the bell peppers with the quinoa mixture and place them in a baking dish.
6. Top each pepper with shredded cheese.
7. Cover with foil and bake for 30 minutes. Remove the foil and bake for another 10 minutes until the cheese is bubbly and slightly browned.
8. Serve hot.

Nutrition Info Per Serving (Serves 4):

- Calories: 350
- Fat: 12g
- Carbohydrates: 50g
- Protein: 15g
- Sodium: 600mg

Cooking Time:

- Preparation time: 20 minutes
- Cooking time: 40 minutes
- Total time: 60 minutes

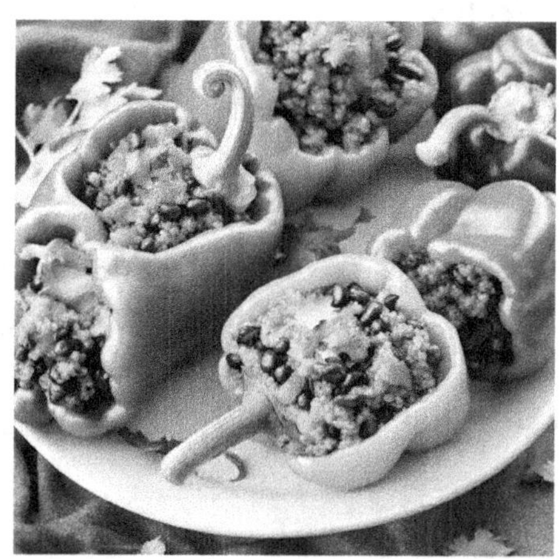

24. Grilled Asparagus with Lemon Tarragon Dressing

Ingredients:

- 1 lb asparagus, trimmed
- 2 tbsp olive oil
- Salt and pepper to taste
- For the dressing:
  - Juice of 1 lemon
  - 1 tbsp fresh tarragon, chopped
  - 1/3 cup olive oil
  - Salt and pepper to taste

Instructions:

1. Preheat your grill to medium-high heat.
2. Toss the asparagus with 2 tbsp olive oil and season with salt and pepper.
3. Grill the asparagus for about 3-4 minutes on each side, until tender and charred.
4. For the dressing, whisk together lemon juice, chopped tarragon, 1/3 cup olive oil, and season with salt and pepper.
5. Drizzle the dressing over the grilled asparagus before serving.

Nutrition Info Per Serving (Serves 4):

- Calories: 220
- Fat: 21g
- Carbohydrates: 5g
- Protein: 3g
- Sodium: 50mg

Cooking Time:

- Preparation time: 10 minutes
- Cooking time: 8 minutes
- Total time: 18 minutes

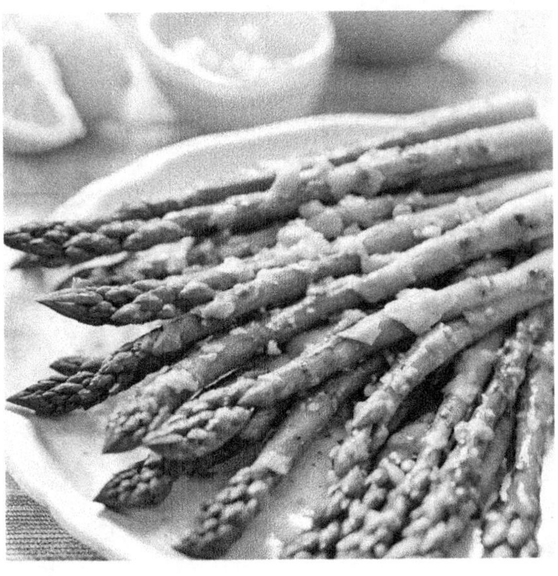

Fish Recipes

1. Grilled Salmon with Lemon Herb Marinade
Ingredients:
- 4 salmon fillets (6 oz each)
- 2 lemons, juiced and zested
- 2 cloves garlic, minced
- 2 tbsp olive oil
- 1 tbsp fresh dill, chopped
- 1 tbsp fresh parsley, chopped
- Salt and pepper to taste

Instructions:
1. In a small bowl, whisk together lemon juice, lemon zest, garlic, olive oil, dill, parsley, salt, and pepper.
2. Place salmon fillets in a shallow dish or resealable plastic bag. Pour the marinade over the salmon, ensuring each fillet is well coated. Refrigerate for at least 30 minutes.
3. Preheat grill to medium-high heat.
4. Remove salmon from marinade, letting excess drip off. Grill each fillet for 4-5 minutes per side, or until the fish flakes easily with a fork.
5. Serve the grilled salmon with additional lemon wedges on the side.

Nutrition Info Per Serving (Serves 4):
- Calories: 280
- Fat: 18g
- Carbohydrates: 2g
- Protein: 28g
- Sodium: 75mg

Cooking Time:
- Preparation time: 10 minutes (plus 30 minutes for marinating)
- Cooking time: 10 minutes
- Total time: 50 minutes

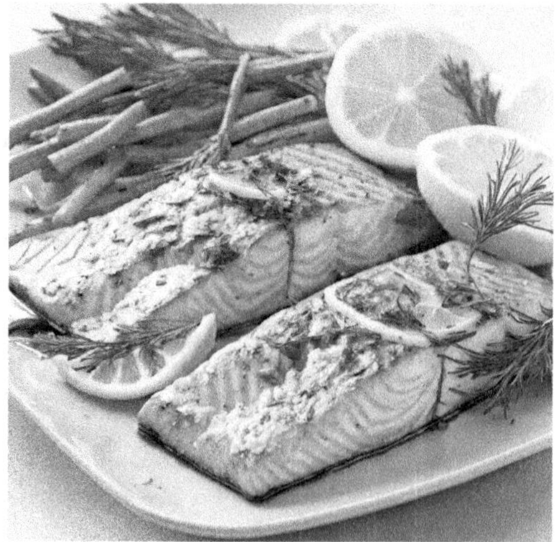

2. Shrimp Stir-Fry with Mixed Vegetables

Ingredients:

- 1 lb shrimp, peeled and deveined
- 2 cups broccoli florets
- 1 red bell pepper, sliced
- 1 yellow bell pepper, sliced
- 1 carrot, julienned
- 2 tbsp soy sauce
- 1 tbsp sesame oil
- 1 tbsp ginger, minced
- 2 cloves garlic, minced
- 1 tbsp olive oil
- Salt and pepper to taste

Instructions:

1. Heat olive oil in a large skillet or wok over medium-high heat.
2. Add garlic and ginger, and sauté for 30 seconds.
3. Add shrimp and cook for 2-3 minutes until pink and nearly cooked through. Remove shrimp and set aside.
4. In the same skillet, add broccoli, bell peppers, and carrots. Stir-fry for about 5 minutes, or until vegetables are tender-crisp.
5. Return shrimp to the skillet. Add soy sauce and sesame oil, and stir to combine. Cook for another 2 minutes.
6. Season with salt and pepper to taste.
7. Serve hot.

Nutrition Info Per Serving (Serves 4):

- Calories: 220
- Fat: 8g
- Carbohydrates: 10g
- Protein: 25g
- Sodium: 480mg

Cooking Time:

- Preparation time: 10 minutes
- Cooking time: 10 minutes
- Total time: 20 minutes

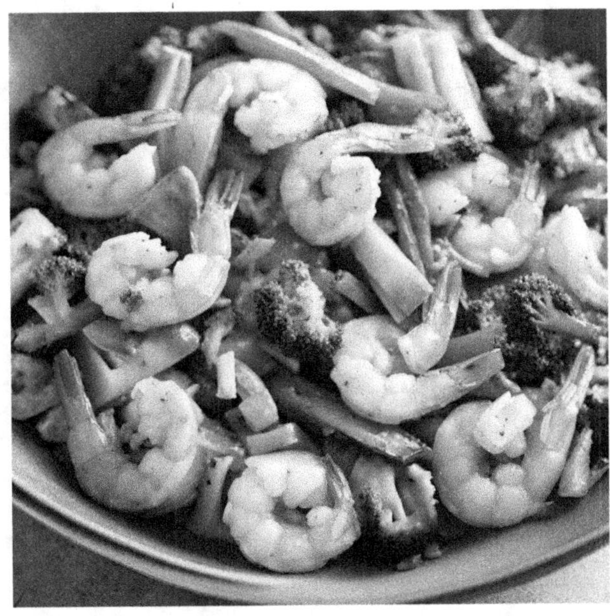

3. Baked Cod with Olive Tapenade

Ingredients:

- 4 cod fillets (6 oz each)
- 1/2 cup olives, pitted and chopped
- 2 tbsp capers, rinsed and chopped
- 2 cloves garlic, minced
- 1 lemon, zested
- 2 tbsp olive oil
- Salt and pepper to taste
- Fresh parsley, chopped for garnish

Instructions:

1. Preheat the oven to 400°F (200°C).
2. In a small bowl, mix together olives, capers, garlic, lemon zest, and 1 tbsp olive oil.
3. Place cod fillets in a baking dish. Season each fillet with salt and pepper.
4. Spoon the olive tapenade evenly over the top of each fillet.
5. Drizzle with the remaining olive oil.
6. Bake in the preheated oven for 12-15 minutes, or until fish flakes easily with a fork.
7. Garnish with fresh parsley before serving.

Nutrition Info Per Serving (Serves 4):

- Calories: 230
- Fat: 10g
- Carbohydrates: 2g
- Protein: 30g
- Sodium: 300mg

Cooking Time:

- Preparation time: 10 minutes
- Cooking time: 15 minutes
- Total time: 25 minutes

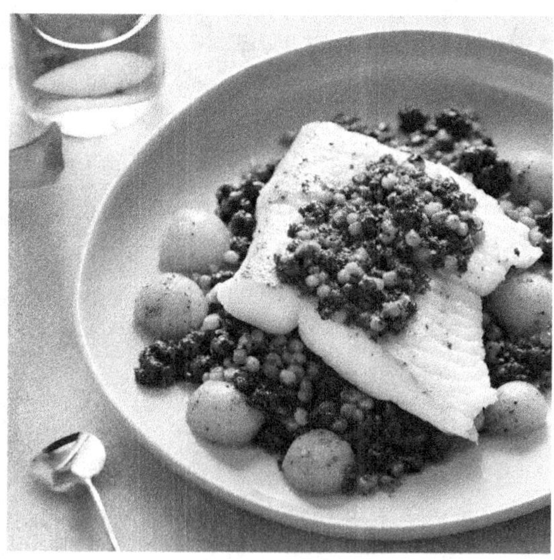

4. Pan-Seared Trout with Walnut Gremolata

Ingredients:

- 4 trout fillets (6 oz each)
- 1/2 cup walnuts, finely chopped
- 2 cloves garlic, minced
- Zest of 1 lemon
- 2 tbsp parsley, finely chopped
- 2 tbsp olive oil
- Salt and pepper to taste

Instructions:

1. In a small bowl, combine walnuts, garlic, lemon zest, and parsley to make the gremolata.
2. Season trout fillets with salt and pepper.
3. Heat olive oil in a large skillet over medium-high heat.
4. Place trout fillets skin-side down in the skillet. Cook for 3-4 minutes until the skin is crispy.
5. Flip the fillets and cook for an additional 2-3 minutes, or until the flesh is opaque and flakes easily with a fork.
6. Serve the trout topped with the walnut gremolata.

Nutrition Info Per Serving (Serves 4):

- Calories: 320
- Fat: 22g
- Carbohydrates: 2g
- Protein: 28g
- Sodium: 75mg

Cooking Time:

- Preparation time: 10 minutes
- Cooking time: 7 minutes
- Total time: 17 minutes

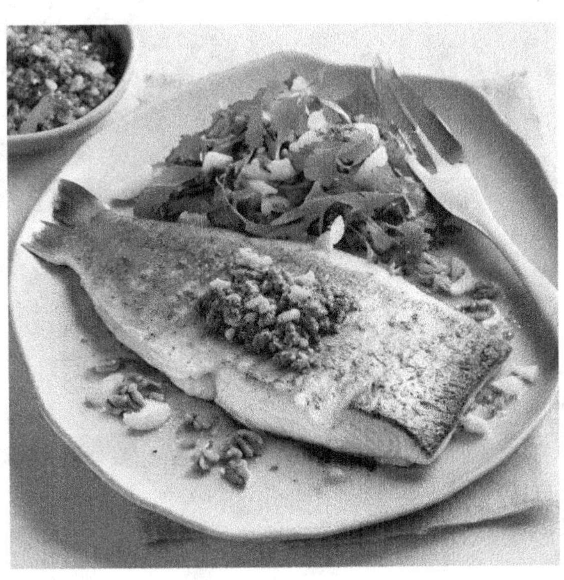

5. Sea Bass with Mango Salsa

Ingredients:

- 4 sea bass fillets (6 oz each)
- 1 mango, diced
- 1 red bell pepper, diced
- 1/2 red onion, diced
- Juice of 1 lime
- 1 tbsp chopped cilantro
- Salt and pepper to taste
- 2 tbsp olive oil

Instructions:

1. Preheat the oven to 400°F (200°C).
2. Season sea bass fillets with salt and pepper.
3. Heat olive oil in a skillet over medium-high heat. Sear the fillets for 2 minutes on each side.
4. Transfer the fillets to a baking dish and bake for 10 minutes, or until the fish flakes easily with a fork.
5. In a bowl, combine mango, red bell pepper, red onion, lime juice, and cilantro to make the salsa. Season with salt to taste.
6. Serve the baked sea bass topped with mango salsa.

Nutrition Info Per Serving (Serves 4):

- Calories: 280
- Fat: 12g
- Carbohydrates: 12g
- Protein: 34g
- Sodium: 75mg

Cooking Time:

- Preparation time: 15 minutes
- Cooking time: 12 minutes
- Total time: 27 minutes

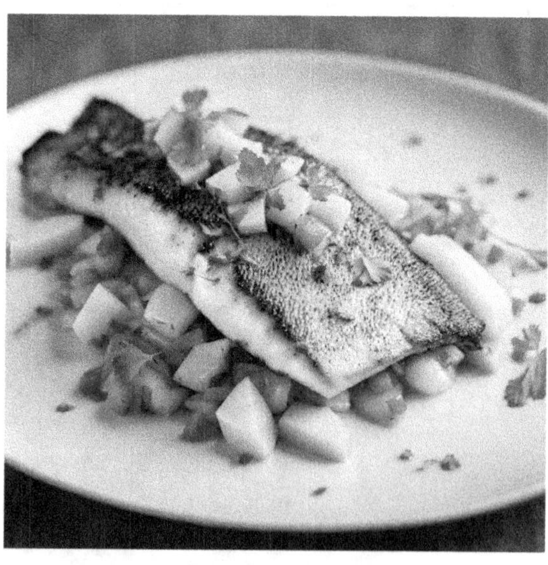

6. Mussels in White Wine and Garlic Sauce

Ingredients:

- 2 lbs mussels, cleaned and de-bearded
- 1 cup dry white wine
- 3 cloves garlic, minced
- 1/4 cup chopped parsley
- 2 tbsp butter
- 1 shallot, minced
- Fresh ground pepper to taste

Instructions:

1. In a large pot, melt butter over medium heat. Add shallot and garlic, and sauté until translucent.
2. Add white wine and bring to a simmer.
3. Add the mussels and cover the pot. Cook for 5-7 minutes, or until all mussels have opened (discard any that do not open).
4. Stir in chopped parsley and season with fresh ground pepper.
5. Serve hot with the broth.

Nutrition Info Per Serving (Serves 4):

- Calories: 240
- Fat: 8g
- Carbohydrates: 10g
- Protein: 25g
- Sodium: 290mg

Cooking Time:

- Preparation time: 10 minutes
- Cooking time: 10 minutes
- Total time: 20 minutes

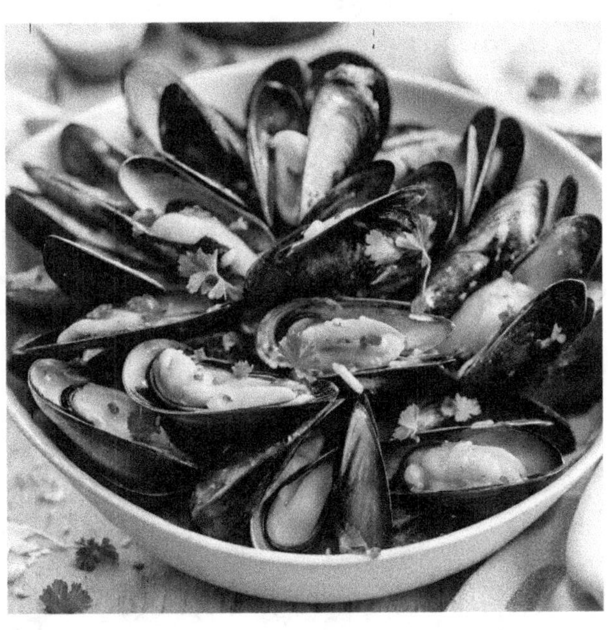

7. Tilapia in Parchment with Tomatoes and Olives

Ingredients:

- 4 tilapia fillets (6 oz each)
- 1 cup cherry tomatoes, halved
- 1/2 cup Kalamata olives, pitted and halved
- 4 sprigs fresh thyme
- 4 tsp olive oil
- Salt and pepper to taste
- Parchment paper

Instructions:

1. Preheat the oven to 400°F (200°C).
2. Cut four large pieces of parchment paper. Place a tilapia fillet in the center of each piece.
3. Top each fillet with equal amounts of tomatoes, olives, and a sprig of thyme. Drizzle with 1 tsp olive oil each, and season with salt and pepper.
4. Fold the parchment paper over the fish, twisting the edges to seal.
5. Place the packets on a baking sheet and bake for 12-15 minutes, until the fish is cooked through.
6. Serve the packets sealed, allowing guests to open them.

Nutrition Info Per Serving (Serves 4):

- Calories: 220
- Fat: 10g
- Carbohydrates: 6g
- Protein: 26g
- Sodium: 300mg

Cooking Time:

- Preparation time: 10 minutes
- Cooking time: 15 minutes
- Total time: 25 minutes

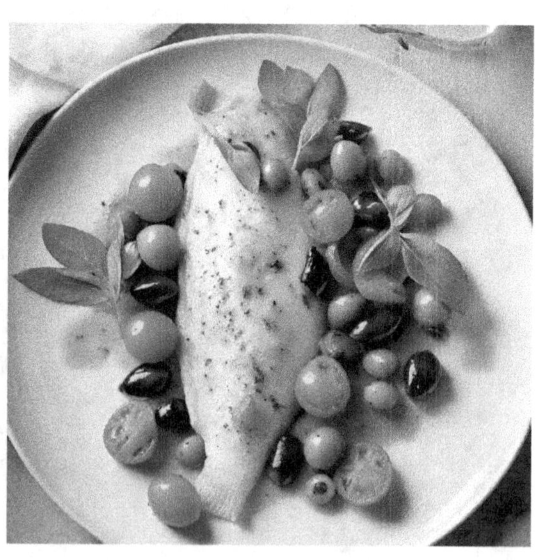

8. Clam Chowder with Corn and Potatoes

Ingredients:

- 2 cups chopped clams, drained with juice reserved
- 2 cups diced potatoes
- 1 cup corn kernels
- 1 onion, diced
- 2 celery stalks, diced
- 2 cups vegetable broth
- 1 cup heavy cream
- 2 tbsp butter
- 2 tbsp flour
- Salt and pepper to taste
- Fresh parsley, chopped for garnish

Instructions:

1. In a large pot, melt butter over medium heat. Add onion and celery, and sauté until softened.
2. Stir in flour to form a roux. Gradually add the vegetable broth and reserved clam juice, stirring continuously.
3. Add potatoes and bring to a boil. Reduce heat and simmer until potatoes are tender, about 15 minutes.
4. Stir in clams and corn, and cook for another 5 minutes.
5. Reduce heat to low and stir in heavy cream. Season with salt and pepper.
6. Heat gently, making sure not to boil, for another 5 minutes.
7. Serve hot, garnished with fresh parsley.

Nutrition Info Per Serving (Serves 4):

- Calories: 350
- Fat: 18g
- Carbohydrates: 35g
- Protein: 15g
- Sodium: 300mg

Cooking Time:

- Preparation time: 15 minutes
- Cooking time: 30 minutes
- Total time: 45 minutes

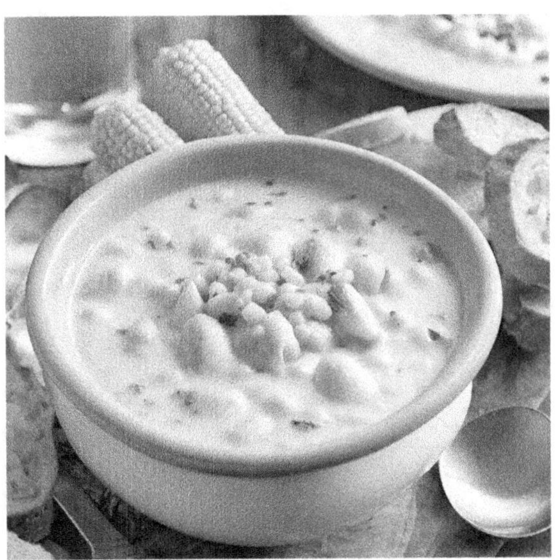

9. Herb-Rubbed Tuna Steak

Ingredients:

- 4 tuna steaks (6 oz each)
- 2 tbsp olive oil
- 1 tbsp dried basil
- 1 tbsp dried oregano
- 1 tsp garlic powder
- Salt and pepper to taste

Instructions:

1. In a small bowl, mix together basil, oregano, garlic powder, salt, and pepper.
2. Rub each tuna steak with olive oil and then coat with the herb mixture.
3. Heat a grill or skillet to medium-high heat. Grill the tuna steaks for 2-3 minutes per side for medium-rare, or until desired doneness is reached.
4. Serve immediately, garnished with a lemon wedge.

Nutrition Info Per Serving (Serves 4):

- Calories: 280
- Fat: 10g
- Carbohydrates: 1g
- Protein: 40g
- Sodium: 75mg

Cooking Time:

- Preparation time: 10 minutes
- Cooking time: 6 minutes
- Total time: 16 minutes

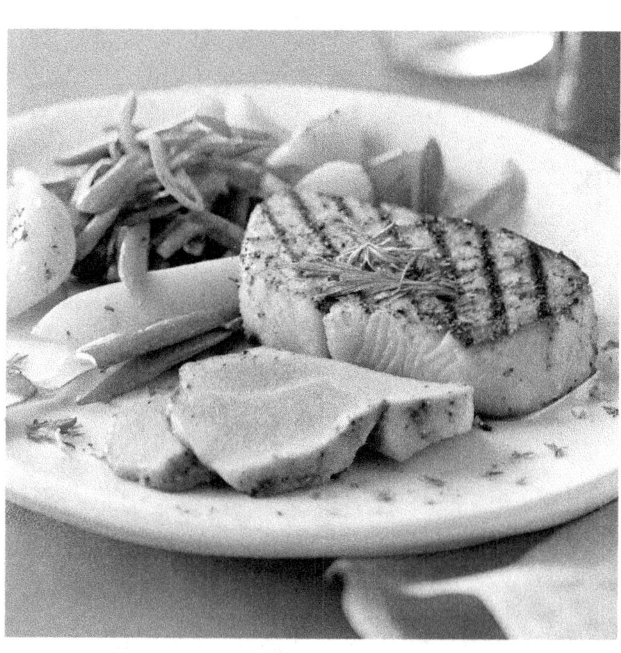

10. Ceviche with Shrimp and Avocado

Ingredients:

- 1 lb raw shrimp, peeled and deveined
- 4 limes, juiced
- 1 orange, juiced
- 1 red onion, finely chopped
- 1 avocado, diced
- 1/4 cup chopped cilantro
- 1 jalapeño, seeded and finely chopped
- Salt to taste

Instructions:

1. Chop the shrimp into 1/2-inch pieces and place in a large bowl.
2. Add lime juice and orange juice so that the shrimp are submerged. Let marinate in the refrigerator for about 2-3 hours, until shrimp are opaque and "cooked" in the acid.
3. Drain the shrimp and discard the marinade.
4. Mix in red onion, avocado, cilantro, and jalapeño. Season with salt.
5. Serve chilled, garnished with extra lime wedges.

Nutrition Info Per Serving (Serves 4):

- Calories: 220
- Fat: 9g
- Carbohydrates: 12g
- Protein: 24g
- Sodium: 150mg

Cooking Time:

- Preparation time: 15 minutes (plus 2-3 hours marinating)
- Total time: 2 hours 30 minutes

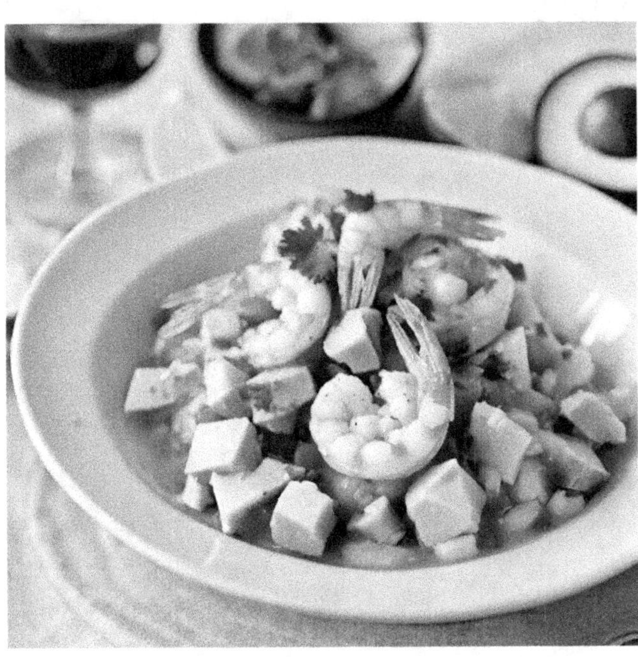

11. Smoked Haddock with Pea Puree

Ingredients:

- 4 smoked haddock fillets (about 6 oz each)
- 2 cups frozen peas
- 1/4 cup milk
- 2 tbsp butter
- Salt and pepper to taste
- Fresh mint leaves, for garnish

Instructions:

1. In a saucepan, bring water to a boil and gently poach the haddock fillets for about 5-7 minutes or until cooked through. Remove and keep warm.
2. In another saucepan, cook the peas in boiling water for about 3 minutes, then drain.
3. Blend the peas with milk and butter in a food processor until smooth. Season with salt and pepper.
4. Serve the smoked haddock on a bed of pea puree, garnished with fresh mint leaves.

Nutrition Info Per Serving (Serves 4):

- Calories: 280
- Fat: 9g
- Carbohydrates: 15g
- Protein: 35g
- Sodium: 580mg

Cooking Time:

- Preparation time: 10 minutes
- Cooking time: 15 minutes
- Total time: 25 minutes

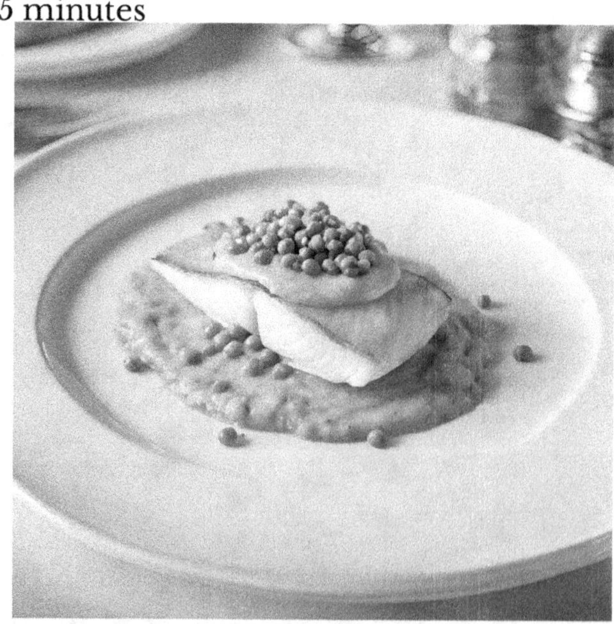

12. Grilled Octopus with Lemon and Parsley

Ingredients:

- 1 large octopus, cleaned (about 2-3 lbs)
- 1/4 cup olive oil
- Juice of 2 lemons
- 1/4 cup chopped parsley
- 2 cloves garlic, minced
- Salt and pepper to taste

Instructions:

1. In a large pot, boil the octopus for about 45-60 minutes until tender. Drain and let cool.
2. Once cool, cut the tentacles and toss them with olive oil, lemon juice, garlic, salt, and pepper.
3. Preheat the grill to medium-high heat. Grill the octopus pieces for about 2-3 minutes on each side until charred and crispy.
4. Garnish with chopped parsley and serve with additional lemon wedges.

Nutrition Info Per Serving (Serves 4):

- Calories: 300
- Fat: 14g
- Carbohydrates: 8g
- Protein: 35g
- Sodium: 450mg

Cooking Time:

- Preparation time: 20 minutes (plus boiling time)
- Cooking time: 6 minutes
- Total time: 1 hour 26 minutes

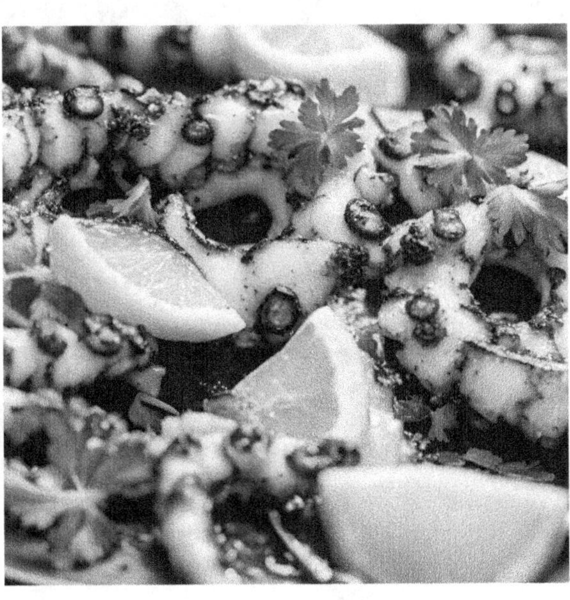

13. Fish Tacos with Cabbage Slaw

Ingredients:

- 1 lb white fish fillets (such as cod or tilapia)
- 8 small corn tortillas
- 2 cups shredded cabbage
- 1 carrot, julienned
- 1/4 cup cilantro, chopped
- 1/4 cup sour cream
- 1 lime, juiced
- 2 tbsp olive oil
- 1 tsp chili powder
- Salt and pepper to taste

Instructions:

1. Preheat a skillet over medium-high heat. Rub the fish with olive oil, chili powder, salt, and pepper.
2. Cook the fish for about 4 minutes per side or until cooked through. Break into flakes.
3. In a bowl, mix the cabbage, carrot, cilantro, and lime juice. Season with salt and pepper.
4. Warm the tortillas on the grill or in a skillet.
5. Assemble the tacos by placing fish flakes and slaw into each tortilla.
6. Top with a dollop of sour cream and serve immediately.

Nutrition Info Per Serving (Serves 4):

- Calories: 320
- Fat: 15g
- Carbohydrates: 28g
- Protein: 20g
- Sodium: 150mg

Cooking Time:

- Preparation time: 15 minutes
- Cooking time: 8 minutes
- Total time: 23 minutes

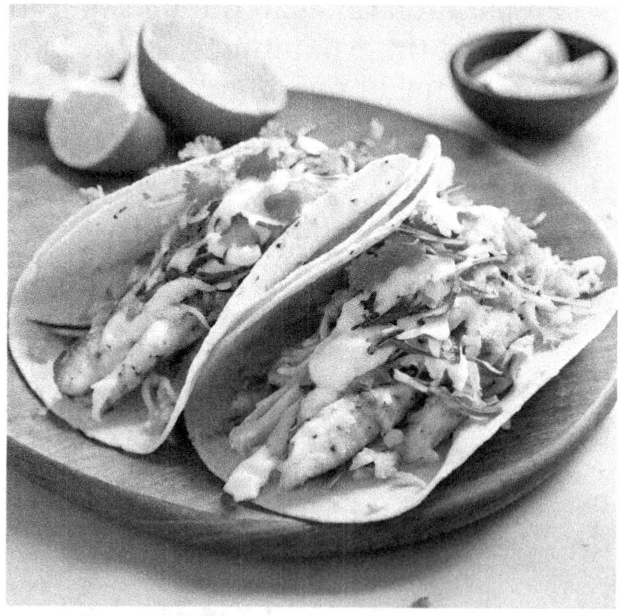

14. Lobster Salad with Citrus Vinaigrette

Ingredients:

- 4 lobster tails, cooked and meat removed
- 1/4 cup olive oil
- Juice of 1 orange
- Juice of 1 lemon
- 1 tsp honey
- 1 tsp mustard
- 1/4 cup mixed greens (such as arugula and spinach)
- 1 avocado, diced
- Salt and pepper to taste

Instructions:

1. In a small bowl, whisk together olive oil, orange juice, lemon juice, honey, and mustard to make the vinaigrette. Season with salt and pepper.
2. Slice the lobster meat and place it in a large mixing bowl.
3. Add the mixed greens and diced avocado.
4. Drizzle the vinaigrette over the salad and gently toss to combine.
5. Serve chilled.

Nutrition Info Per Serving (Serves 4):

- Calories: 320
- Fat: 22g
- Carbohydrates: 12g
- Protein: 20g
- Sodium: 180mg

Cooking Time:

- Preparation time: 15 minutes
- Total time: 15 minutes

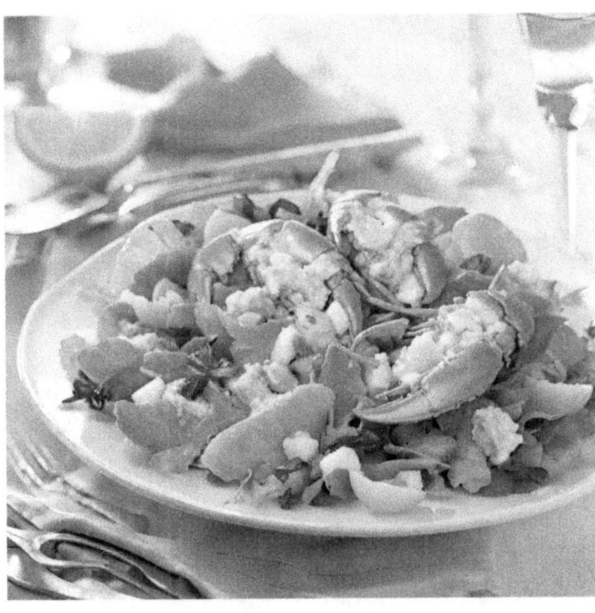

15. Seared Scallops with Butternut Squash Puree
Ingredients:

- 12 large sea scallops
- 2 cups butternut squash, cubed
- 1/4 cup milk
- 2 tbsp butter
- Salt and pepper to taste
- Olive oil for searing
- Fresh thyme for garnish

Instructions:

1. Steam or boil the butternut squash until tender, about 15-20 minutes. Drain and puree in a blender with milk and 1 tablespoon of butter until smooth. Season with salt and pepper.
2. Pat scallops dry with paper towels. Season with salt and pepper.
3. Heat olive oil in a skillet over high heat. Add scallops; sear for about 1-2 minutes on each side until a golden crust forms.
4. Serve scallops over butternut squash puree and garnish with fresh thyme.

Nutrition Info Per Serving (Serves 4):

- Calories: 250
- Fat: 10g
- Carbohydrates: 20g
- Protein: 20g
- Sodium: 480mg

Cooking Time:

- Preparation time: 20 minutes
- Cooking time: 25 minutes
- Total time: 45 minutes

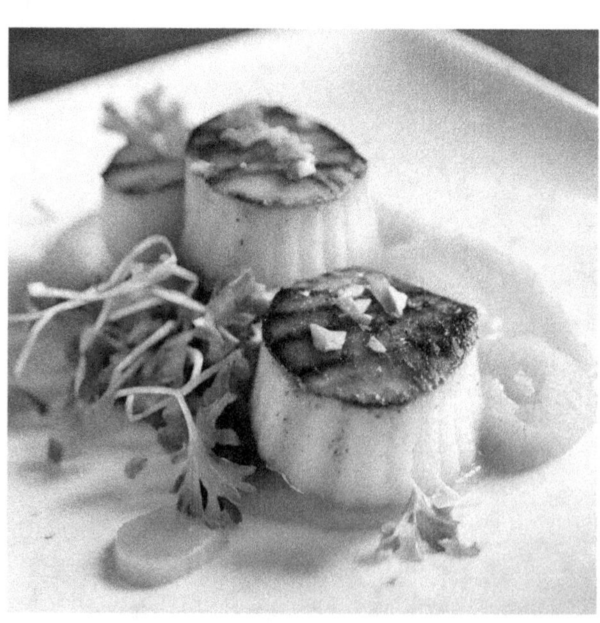

16. Salmon Poke Bowl

Ingredients:

- 1 lb sushi-grade salmon, cubed
- 2 cups cooked brown rice
- 1 avocado, diced
- 1/2 cucumber, sliced
- 1/4 cup soy sauce
- 1 tsp sesame oil
- 1 tsp honey
- 2 tbsp scallions, chopped
- 1 tbsp sesame seeds
- 1 nori sheet, shredded

Instructions:

1. In a bowl, mix soy sauce, sesame oil, and honey. Add cubed salmon and marinate for about 15 minutes in the refrigerator.
2. Assemble the poke bowl with a base of brown rice. Top with marinated salmon, diced avocado, sliced cucumber, and shredded nori.
3. Sprinkle with scallions and sesame seeds.
4. Serve immediately.

Nutrition Info Per Serving (Serves 4):

- Calories: 420
- Fat: 18g
- Carbohydrates: 35g
- Protein: 30g
- Sodium: 800mg

Cooking Time:

- Preparation time: 20 minutes
- Total time: 20 minutes

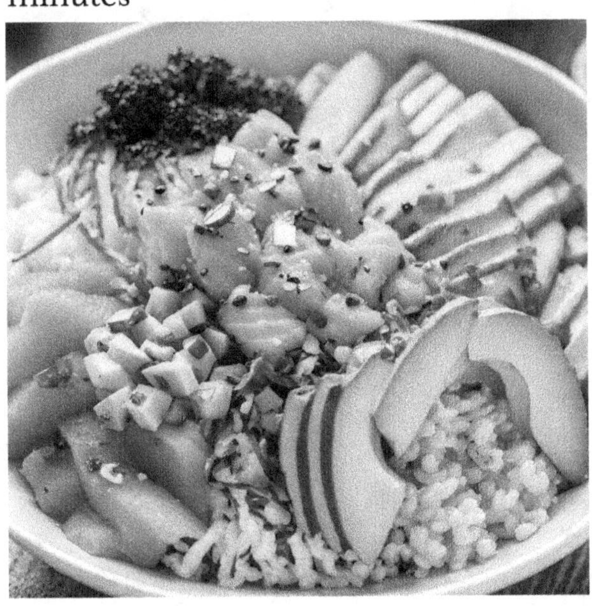

17. Catfish Étouffée

Ingredients:

- 4 catfish fillets, cut into chunks
- 1 onion, chopped
- 1 green bell pepper, chopped
- 2 celery stalks, chopped
- 3 cloves garlic, minced
- 1 cup seafood or chicken broth
- 1/4 cup all-purpose flour
- 1/4 cup vegetable oil
- 2 tbsp Cajun seasoning
- Salt and pepper to taste
- Fresh parsley, chopped for garnish

Instructions:

1. Heat oil in a large skillet over medium heat. Add flour to make a roux, stirring continuously until it turns a golden brown color.
2. Add onion, bell pepper, celery, and garlic to the roux, and cook until vegetables are soft.
3. Stir in broth gradually, then add Cajun seasoning, salt, and pepper.
4. Add catfish chunks, cover, and simmer for about 10-15 minutes until fish is cooked through.
5. Garnish with fresh parsley and serve hot over rice.

Nutrition Info Per Serving (Serves 4):

- Calories: 330
- Fat: 15g
- Carbohydrates: 15g
- Protein: 35g
- Sodium: 600mg

Cooking Time:

- Preparation time: 15 minutes
- Cooking time: 25 minutes
- Total time: 40 minutes

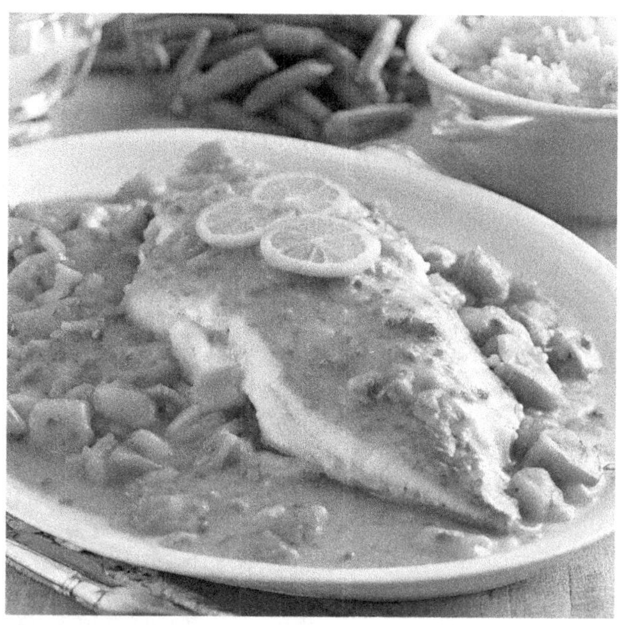

18. Garlic Butter Shrimp Skewers

Ingredients:

- 1 lb large shrimp, peeled and deveined
- 3 cloves garlic, minced
- 4 tbsp butter, melted
- 1 lemon, juiced
- Salt and pepper to taste
- Fresh parsley, chopped for garnish
- Wooden or metal skewers

Instructions:

1. In a bowl, combine melted butter, garlic, lemon juice, salt, and pepper.
2. Thread the shrimp onto skewers.
3. Brush the shrimp generously with the garlic butter mixture.
4. Preheat a grill or grill pan over medium-high heat.
5. Grill the shrimp skewers for 2-3 minutes on each side or until shrimp are pink and opaque.
6. Garnish with chopped parsley and serve immediately.

Nutrition Info Per Serving (Serves 4):

- Calories: 200
- Fat: 12g
- Carbohydrates: 2g
- Protein: 20g
- Sodium: 210mg

Cooking Time:

- Preparation time: 10 minutes
- Cooking time: 6 minutes
- Total time: 16 minutes

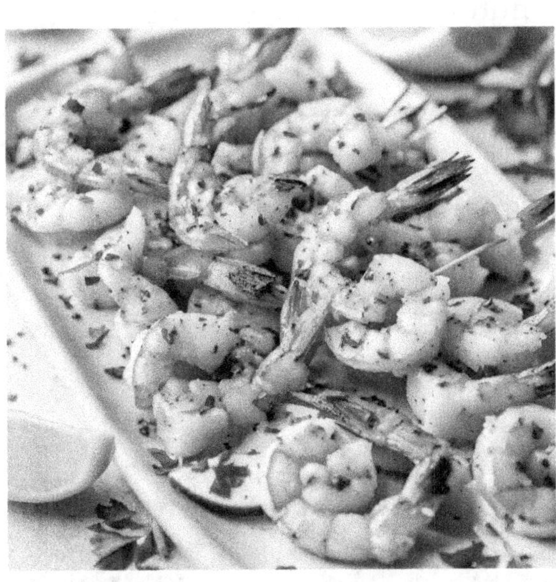

19. Baked Lemon Sole with Capers

Ingredients:

- 4 sole fillets (about 6 oz each)
- 2 lemons, juiced and zested
- 2 tbsp capers, rinsed
- 2 tbsp olive oil
- Salt and pepper to taste
- Fresh dill, chopped for garnish

Instructions:

1. Preheat the oven to 375°F (190°C).
2. Place sole fillets in a baking dish.
3. In a small bowl, mix together lemon juice, lemon zest, capers, and olive oil.
4. Pour the mixture over the sole fillets and season with salt and pepper.
5. Bake in the preheated oven for 12-15 minutes, until the fish flakes easily with a fork.
6. Garnish with fresh dill and serve immediately.

Nutrition Info Per Serving (Serves 4):

- Calories: 220
- Fat: 10g
- Carbohydrates: 3g
- Protein: 30g
- Sodium: 320mg

Cooking Time:

- Preparation time: 10 minutes
- Cooking time: 15 minutes
- Total time: 25 minutes

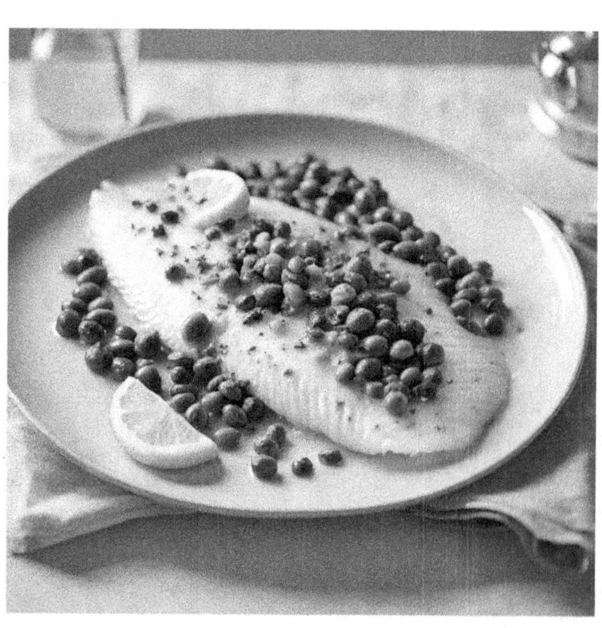

20. Scallop and Chorizo Pasta

Ingredients:

- 1 lb scallops
- 6 oz chorizo, sliced
- 12 oz pasta (such as linguine or spaghetti)
- 2 cloves garlic, minced
- 1/4 cup white wine
- 2 tbsp olive oil
- Salt and pepper to taste
- Fresh parsley, chopped for garnish

Instructions:

1. Cook pasta according to package instructions until al dente. Drain and set aside.
2. Heat olive oil in a large skillet over medium heat. Add chorizo and fry until crispy.
3. Add garlic and scallops to the skillet. Cook scallops for about 2 minutes per side or until golden and opaque.
4. Deglaze the pan with white wine and let reduce slightly.
5. Toss the cooked pasta with the scallop and chorizo mixture. Season with salt and pepper.
6. Garnish with fresh parsley and serve immediately.

Nutrition Info Per Serving (Serves 4):

- Calories: 580
- Fat: 22g
- Carbohydrates: 58g
- Protein: 36g
- Sodium: 820mg

Cooking Time:

- Preparation time: 10 minutes
- Cooking time: 20 minutes
- Total time: 30 minutes

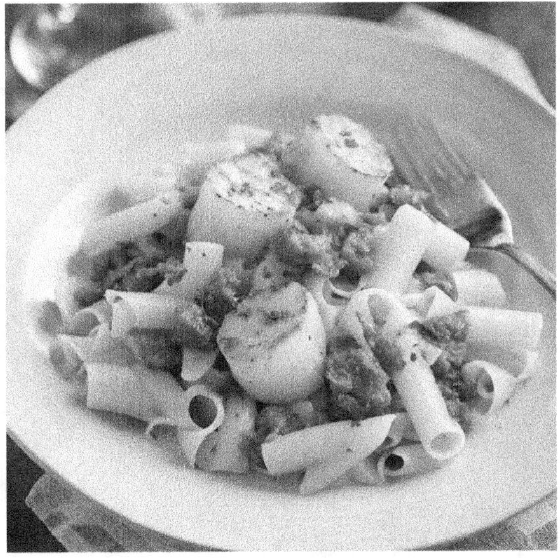

21. Pan-Fried Sardines with Lemon Aioli

Ingredients:

- 1 lb fresh sardines, cleaned and gutted
- 1 cup all-purpose flour
- 2 lemons, one juiced and one sliced
- 1/2 cup mayonnaise
- 1 clove garlic, minced
- Salt and pepper to taste
- Olive oil for frying
- Fresh parsley, chopped for garnish

Instructions:

1. Season the sardines with salt and pepper, then dredge in flour, shaking off the excess.
2. Heat olive oil in a skillet over medium-high heat. Pan-fry the sardines for 2-3 minutes on each side until crispy and golden. Remove and drain on paper towels.
3. For the aioli, mix mayonnaise, lemon juice, minced garlic, and a pinch of salt in a small bowl.
4. Serve the sardines with lemon aioli, garnished with lemon slices and chopped parsley.

Nutrition Info Per Serving (Serves 4):

- Calories: 370
- Fat: 22g
- Carbohydrates: 18g
- Protein: 25g
- Sodium: 340mg

Cooking Time:

- Preparation time: 10 minutes
- Cooking time: 6 minutes
- Total time: 16 minutes

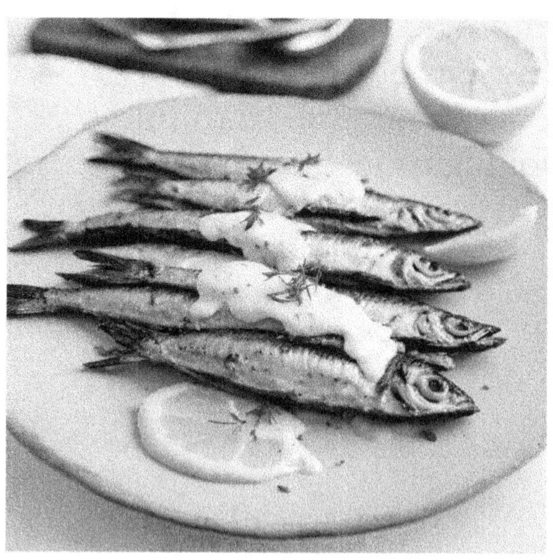

22. Paella with Seafood and Saffron

Ingredients:

- 1 lb mixed seafood (shrimp, mussels, and squid)
- 1 cup arborio rice
- 3 cups chicken or vegetable broth
- 1/2 cup white wine
- 1 onion, chopped
- 1 bell pepper, diced
- 2 cloves garlic, minced
- 1/2 tsp saffron threads
- 1 tsp paprika
- 2 tbsp olive oil
- Salt and pepper to taste
- Fresh parsley, chopped for garnish
- Lemon wedges for serving

Instructions:

1. Heat olive oil in a large skillet or paella pan over medium heat. Sauté onion, bell pepper, and garlic until softened.
2. Add rice, saffron, and paprika, stirring until the rice is well coated.
3. Pour in white wine and let it simmer until it has mostly evaporated.
4. Add broth and bring to a simmer. Cook without stirring for 15 minutes.
5. Add the seafood, gently pushing it into the rice. Cook for an additional 10 minutes or until seafood is cooked and rice is tender.
6. Remove from heat, cover with a cloth, and let sit for 10 minutes.
7. Garnish with parsley and serve with lemon wedges.

Nutrition Info Per Serving (Serves 4):

- Calories: 460
- Fat: 14g
- Carbohydrates: 50g
- Protein: 30g
- Sodium: 780mg

Cooking Time:

- Preparation time: 15 minutes
- Cooking time: 35 minutes
- Total time: 50 minutes

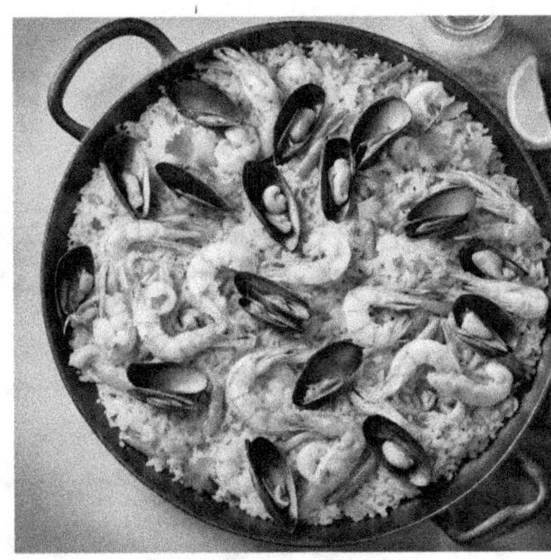

23. Anchovy and Tomato Flatbreads

Ingredients:

- 4 pre-made flatbreads
- 1 can anchovies, drained
- 2 tomatoes, sliced
- 1/4 cup olive oil
- 2 cloves garlic, minced
- Fresh basil leaves
- Salt and pepper to taste

Instructions:

1. Preheat the oven to 400°F (200°C).
2. Brush each flatbread with olive oil and sprinkle minced garlic over them.
3. Arrange tomato slices and anchovies on the flatbreads. Season with salt and pepper.
4. Bake for 10-12 minutes until the edges are crisp and golden.
5. Garnish with fresh basil leaves before serving.

Nutrition Info Per Serving (Serves 4):

- Calories: 330
- Fat: 18g
- Carbohydrates: 32g
- Protein: 12g
- Sodium: 560mg

Cooking Time:

- Preparation time: 10 minutes
- Cooking time: 12 minutes
- Total time: 22 minutes

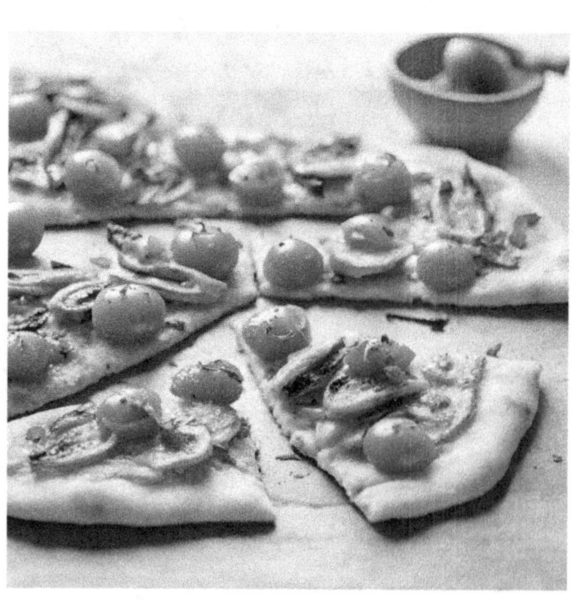

24. Oysters Rockefeller

Ingredients:

- 24 oysters, shucked, on the half shell
- 1/2 cup breadcrumbs
- 1/4 cup grated Parmesan cheese
- 1/2 cup butter, softened
- 2 cloves garlic, minced
- 1/2 cup chopped fresh spinach
- 1/4 cup chopped parsley
- 1 tbsp anise liqueur (optional)
- Salt and pepper to taste
- Lemon wedges for serving

Instructions:

1. Preheat your oven to 450°F (230°C).
2. In a skillet, melt the butter over medium heat. Add garlic and sauté for 1 minute.
3. Stir in spinach and parsley, and cook until the spinach is wilted.
4. Remove from heat and mix in breadcrumbs, Parmesan cheese, anise liqueur (if using), salt, and pepper.
5. Arrange the oysters on a baking sheet. Spoon the spinach mixture on top of each oyster.
6. Bake in the preheated oven for about 10 minutes, until the topping is golden and crispy.
7. Serve hot with lemon wedges on the side.

Nutrition Info Per Serving (Serves 6):

- Calories: 200
- Fat: 15g
- Carbohydrates: 10g
- Protein: 10g
- Sodium: 250mg

Cooking Time:

- Preparation time: 15 minutes
- Cooking time: 10 minutes
- Total time: 25 minutes

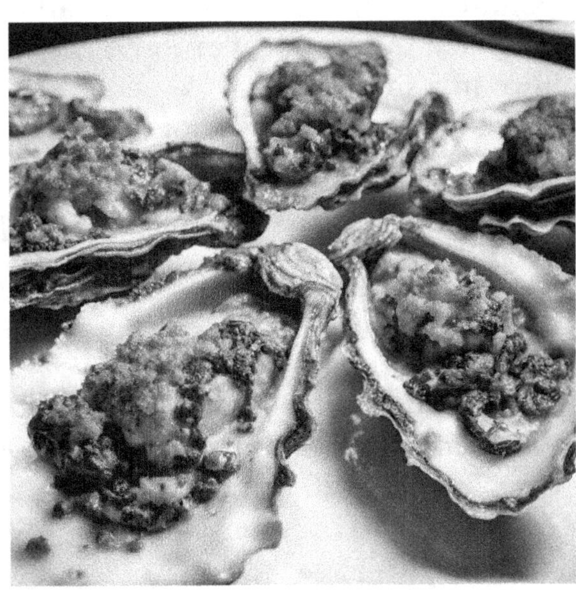

25. Bouillabaisse with Rouille

Ingredients:

- 1 lb mixed fish fillets (such as sea bass, snapper), cut into pieces
- 1/2 lb shrimp, peeled and deveined
- 1/2 lb mussels, cleaned
- 1 onion, chopped
- 1 fennel bulb, thinly sliced
- 3 cloves garlic, minced
- 1 can (14 oz) diced tomatoes
- 4 cups fish stock
- 1/4 cup white wine
- 1 tsp saffron threads
- 1/2 tsp thyme
- Salt and pepper to taste
- For the rouille:
  - 1/2 cup mayonnaise
  - 1 clove garlic, minced
  - 1 tsp paprika
  - Juice of 1/2 lemon

Instructions:

1. In a large pot, heat a little oil over medium heat. Add onion, fennel, and garlic. Cook until softened.
2. Stir in tomatoes, fish stock, white wine, saffron, and thyme. Bring to a simmer.
3. Add the fish, shrimp, and mussels. Cover and cook for about 10 minutes, until the mussels open and the fish is cooked through.
4. To make the rouille, combine mayonnaise, garlic, paprika, and lemon juice in a small bowl.
5. Serve the bouillabaisse hot, topped with a spoonful of rouille.

Nutrition Info Per Serving (Serves 6):

- Calories: 350
- Fat: 18g
- Carbohydrates: 15g
- Protein: 30g
- Sodium: 700mg

Cooking Time:

- Preparation time: 20 minutes
- Cooking time: 20 minutes
- Total time: 40 minutes

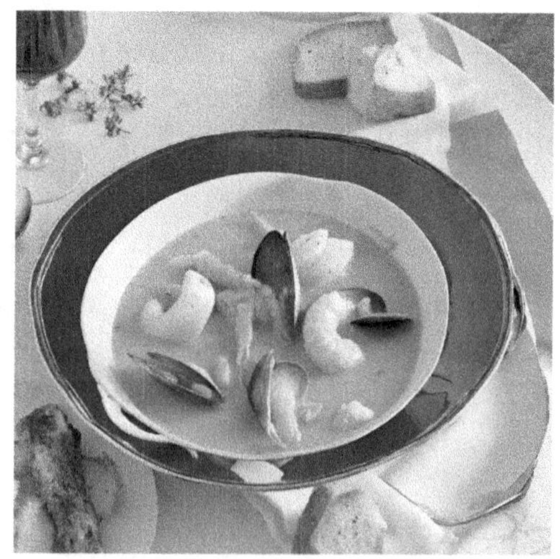

26. Crab-Stuffed Flounder

Ingredients:

- 4 flounder fillets
- 1 cup crabmeat, drained
- 1/4 cup breadcrumbs
- 1/4 cup mayonnaise
- 1 egg
- 1 tbsp chopped parsley
- 1 tsp mustard
- Salt and pepper to taste
- Lemon slices for serving

Instructions:

1. Preheat the oven to 375°F (190°C).
2. In a bowl, mix together crabmeat, breadcrumbs, mayonnaise, egg, parsley, mustard, salt, and pepper.
3. Lay flounder fillets flat on a work surface. Divide the crab mixture among the fillets, placing it on one end of each fillet.
4. Roll up the fillets around the stuffing and secure with toothpicks.
5. Place the stuffed fillets in a baking dish and bake for 20-25 minutes, until the fish is opaque and cooked through.
6. Serve with lemon slices.

Nutrition Info Per Serving (Serves 4):

- Calories: 290
- Fat: 15g
- Carbohydrates: 10g
- Protein: 28g
- Sodium: 380mg

Cooking Time:

- Preparation time: 15 minutes
- Cooking time: 25 minutes
- Total time: 40 minutes

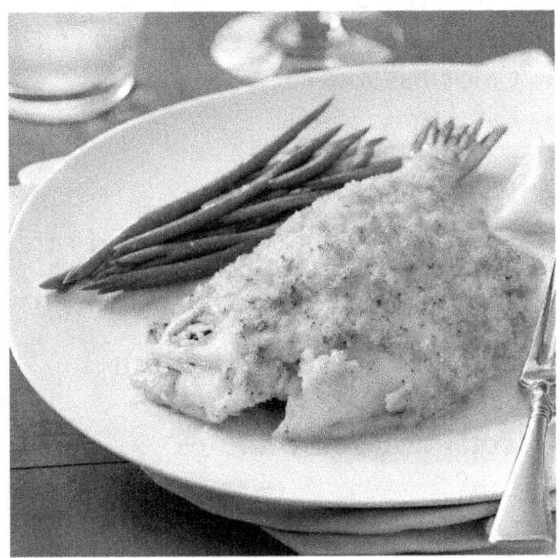

27. Linguine with Clams and White Wine Sauce

Ingredients:

- 1 lb linguine
- 2 lbs fresh clams, cleaned
- 1 cup white wine
- 3 cloves garlic, minced
- 1/4 cup parsley, chopped
- 1/4 cup olive oil
- Red pepper flakes (optional)
- Salt to taste
- Lemon wedges for serving

Instructions:

1. Cook linguine according to package instructions in salted water until al dente. Drain and set aside, reserving 1 cup of pasta water.
2. In a large skillet, heat olive oil over medium heat. Add garlic and sauté until fragrant, about 1 minute. If using, sprinkle in some red pepper flakes for heat.
3. Add the clams to the skillet, along with the white wine. Cover and cook for 5-7 minutes until most clams have opened. Discard any that do not open.
4. Add the cooked linguine to the skillet with the clams. Toss to combine, adding a little reserved pasta water if the mixture seems dry.
5. Season with salt to taste and stir in the chopped parsley.
6. Serve the linguine with clams in bowls, garnished with lemon wedges.

Nutrition Info Per Serving (Serves 4):

- Calories: 560
- Fat: 14g
- Carbohydrates: 70g
- Protein: 30g
- Sodium: 80mg (varies based on the saltiness of the clams and amount of added salt)

Cooking Time:

- Preparation time: 10 minutes
- Cooking time: 20 minutes
- Total time: 30 minutes

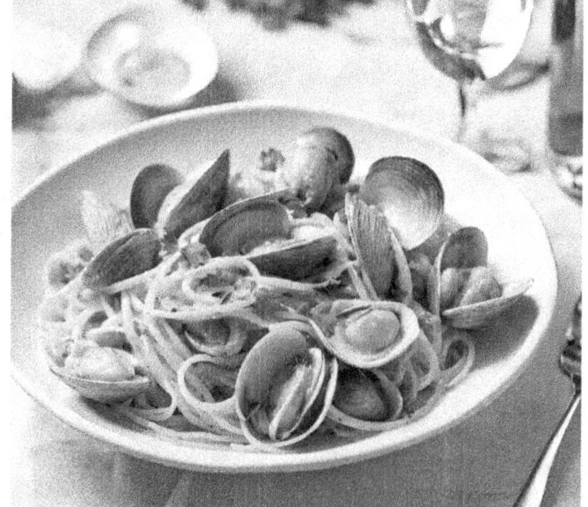

Desserts

1. Hazelnut Gelato

Ingredients:

- 2 cups milk
- 1 cup heavy cream
- 3/4 cup sugar
- 1/2 cup hazelnuts, toasted and finely ground
- 4 egg yolks
- 1 tsp vanilla extract

Instructions:

1. In a saucepan, combine milk, cream, and ground hazelnuts. Heat over medium heat until the mixture just begins to boil. Remove from heat and let steep for 30 minutes. Strain the mixture through a fine-mesh sieve, pressing on the nuts to extract as much liquid as possible.
2. In a separate bowl, whisk together egg yolks and sugar until pale and thick.
3. Slowly whisk the warm hazelnut-infused milk into the egg mixture.
4. Return the mixture to the saucepan and cook over low heat, stirring constantly until the custard thickens and coats the back of a spoon (about 175°F on a thermometer).
5. Remove from heat, stir in vanilla extract, and chill the mixture thoroughly in the refrigerator.
6. Once chilled, churn in an ice cream maker according to the manufacturer's instructions.
7. Freeze until firm, then serve.

Nutrition Info Per Serving (Serves 8):

- Calories: 300
- Fat: 20g
- Carbohydrates: 25g
- Protein: 5g
- Sodium: 50mg

Cooking Time:

- Preparation time: 15 minutes (plus steeping and chilling)
- Cooking time: 10 minutes
- Total time: 25 minutes active, several hours passive

2. Frozen Banana Bites Dipped in Chocolate

Ingredients:

- 3 large bananas
- 1 cup dark chocolate chips
- 1 tbsp coconut oil
- Toppings as desired (chopped nuts, coconut flakes, sprinkles)

Instructions:

1. Peel and slice bananas into 1/2 inch thick slices.
2. Lay banana slices on a baking sheet lined with parchment paper and freeze for at least 2 hours.
3. Melt chocolate chips with coconut oil in a microwave or over a double boiler until smooth.
4. Dip frozen banana slices into melted chocolate, coating them completely. Optionally, sprinkle with toppings.
5. Place the chocolate-covered bananas back on the parchment paper and freeze until the chocolate sets.
6. Serve frozen.

Nutrition Info Per Serving (Serves 6):

- Calories: 210
- Fat: 10g
- Carbohydrates: 30g
- Protein: 2g
- Sodium: 10mg

Cooking Time:

- Preparation time: 10 minutes
- Total time: 2 hours 20 minutes

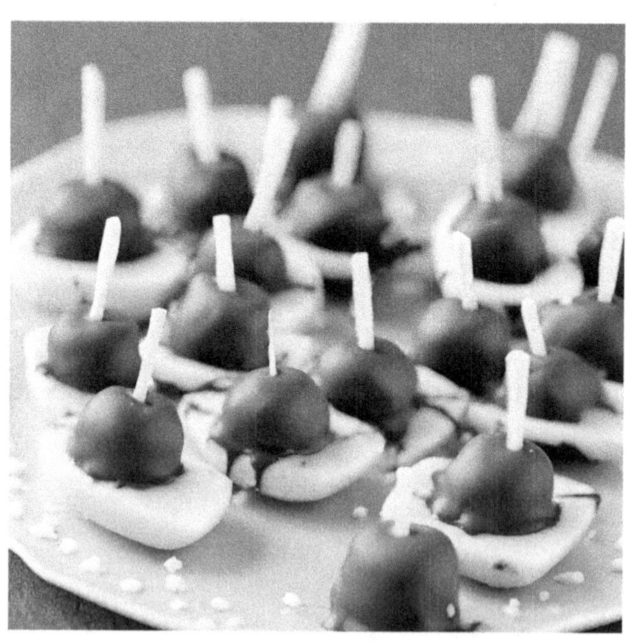

3. Sweet Potato Pie with Marshmallow Meringue

Ingredients:

- For the pie:
    - 1 lb sweet potatoes, peeled and boiled
    - 1/2 cup butter, softened
    - 1 cup sugar
    - 1/2 cup milk
    - 2 eggs
    - 1/2 tsp ground nutmeg
    - 1/2 tsp ground cinnamon
    - 1 tsp vanilla extract
    - 1 (9-inch) unbaked pie crust
- For the meringue:
    - 3 egg whites
    - 1/4 tsp cream of tartar
    - 6 tbsp sugar
    - 1/2 cup mini marshmallows (optional)

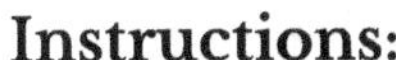

Instructions:

1. Mash boiled sweet potatoes with butter, sugar, milk, eggs, nutmeg, cinnamon, and vanilla until smooth. Pour into the pie crust.
2. Bake in a preheated oven at 350°F (175°C) for 55 minutes, or until a knife inserted in the center comes out clean.
3. For the meringue, beat egg whites and cream of tartar until foamy. Gradually add sugar, continuing to beat until stiff peaks form.
4. Spread meringue over the pie, covering completely. Sprinkle with mini marshmallows if using.
5. Broil for a few minutes until the meringue is golden brown. Watch closely to avoid burning.
6. Serve after cooling.

Nutrition Info Per Serving (Serves 8):

- Calories: 390
- Fat: 18g
- Carbohydrates: 53g
- Protein: 5g
- Sodium: 180mg

Cooking Time:

- Preparation time: 30 minutes
- Cooking time: 55 minutes
- Total time: 1 hour 25 minutes

4. Roasted Stone Fruit with Vanilla Bean
Ingredients:
- 4 peaches, halved and pitted
- 4 plums, halved and pitted
- 2 tbsp honey
- 1 vanilla bean, split lengthwise
- 1/4 cup almond slices, toasted

Instructions:
1. Preheat oven to 375°F (190°C).
2. Arrange fruit halves cut-side up in a baking dish. Drizzle with honey and place the vanilla bean among the fruit.
3. Roast in the oven for 25-30 minutes, or until fruit is tender and juicy.
4. Serve warm, topped with toasted almond slices.

Nutrition Info Per Serving (Serves 4):
- Calories: 150
- Fat: 4g
- Carbohydrates: 27g
- Protein: 2g
- Sodium: 0mg

Cooking Time:
- Preparation time: 10 minutes
- Cooking time: 30 minutes
- Total time: 40 minutes

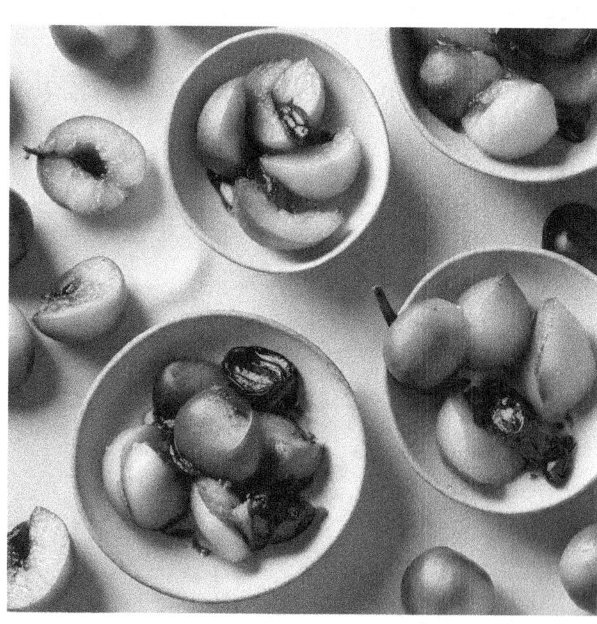

5. Pomegranate and Pistachio Bark

Ingredients:

- 1 lb dark chocolate (70% cocoa or higher), chopped
- 1/2 cup pomegranate seeds
- 1/2 cup shelled pistachios, chopped

Instructions:

1. Line a baking sheet with parchment paper.
2. Melt the chocolate in a heatproof bowl over a pot of simmering water, stirring continuously.
3. Pour the melted chocolate onto the prepared baking sheet, spreading it into an even layer.
4. Sprinkle pomegranate seeds and pistachios evenly over the chocolate.
5. Refrigerate until firm, about 1-2 hours.
6. Break into pieces and serve.

Nutrition Info Per Serving (Serves 8):

- Calories: 320
- Fat: 22g
- Carbohydrates: 25g
- Protein: 4g
- Sodium: 20mg

Cooking Time:

- Preparation time: 10 minutes
- Chilling time: 1-2 hours
- Total time: 1 hour 10 minutes to 2 hours 10 minutes

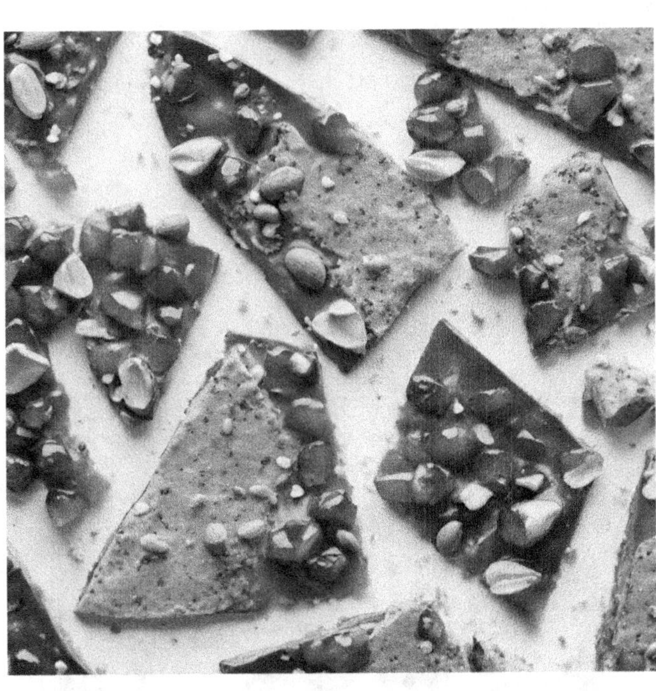

6. Cherry Clafoutis

Ingredients:

- 1 lb fresh cherries, pitted
- 3 eggs
- 1 cup milk
- 1/2 cup all-purpose flour
- 1/3 cup granulated sugar
- 1 tsp vanilla extract
- Powdered sugar for dusting
- Butter for greasing

Instructions:

1. Preheat oven to 350°F (175°C). Grease a 9-inch pie dish with butter.
2. Spread the pitted cherries evenly in the prepared dish.
3. In a blender, combine eggs, milk, flour, sugar, and vanilla extract. Blend until smooth.
4. Pour the batter over the cherries.
5. Bake in the preheated oven for 40-45 minutes, until set and golden brown.
6. Dust with powdered sugar before serving.

Nutrition Info Per Serving (Serves 6):

- Calories: 210
- Fat: 3g
- Carbohydrates: 38g
- Protein: 6g
- Sodium: 50mg

Cooking Time:

- Preparation time: 10 minutes
- Cooking time: 45 minutes
- Total time: 55 minutes

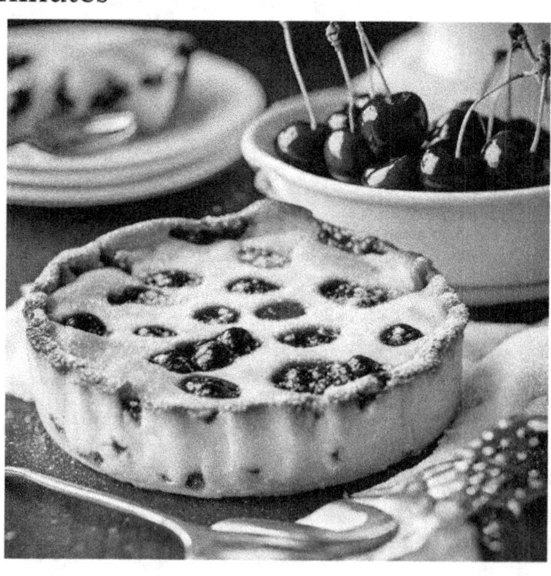

7. Saffron and Cardamom Panna Cotta

Ingredients:

- 2 cups heavy cream
- 1/2 cup sugar
- 1 tsp cardamom, ground
- A pinch of saffron threads
- 1 packet gelatin (about 2 tsp)
- 1/4 cup water

Instructions:

1. In a small bowl, sprinkle gelatin over water and let it soften for about 5 minutes.
2. In a saucepan, heat cream, sugar, cardamom, and saffron just until the mixture starts to simmer. Remove from heat.
3. Add the softened gelatin to the cream mixture and stir until completely dissolved.
4. Pour into molds or ramekins. Refrigerate until set, about 4 hours.
5. Serve chilled.

Nutrition Info Per Serving (Serves 6):

- Calories: 300
- Fat: 22g
- Carbohydrates: 24g
- Protein: 2g
- Sodium: 30mg

Cooking Time:

- Preparation time: 10 minutes
- Chilling time: 4 hours
- Total time: 4 hours 10 minutes

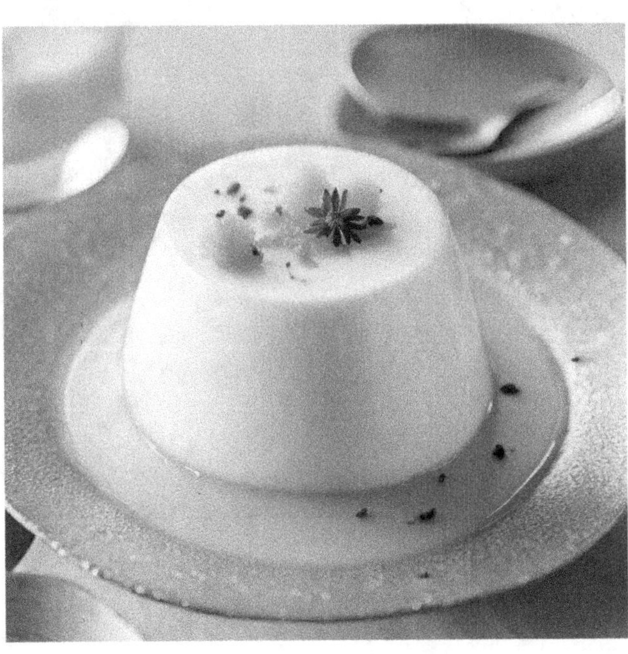

8. Almond and Orange Biscotti

Ingredients:

- 2 cups all-purpose flour
- 3/4 cup sugar
- 1 tsp baking powder
- 1/2 cup almonds, chopped
- Zest of 1 orange
- 2 eggs
- 1/4 cup olive oil
- 1 tsp vanilla extract

Instructions:

1. Preheat oven to 350°F (175°C). Line a baking sheet with parchment paper.
2. In a large bowl, mix flour, sugar, baking powder, almonds, and orange zest.
3. In another bowl, whisk together eggs, olive oil, and vanilla extract. Add to the dry ingredients, mixing until a dough forms.
4. Divide the dough in half and form two logs on the prepared baking sheet.
5. Bake for 25 minutes, then remove from oven and let cool for 10 minutes. Slice diagonally into 1/2-inch thick slices.
6. Return the slices to the baking sheet, cut side down, and bake for an additional 10 minutes on each side, until golden and crisp.
7. Cool on a wire rack.

Nutrition Info Per Serving (Serves 12):

- Calories: 180
- Fat: 7g
- Carbohydrates: 25g
- Protein: 4g
- Sodium: 40mg

Cooking Time:

- Preparation time: 20 minutes
- Cooking time: 45 minutes
- Total time: 1 hour 5 minutes

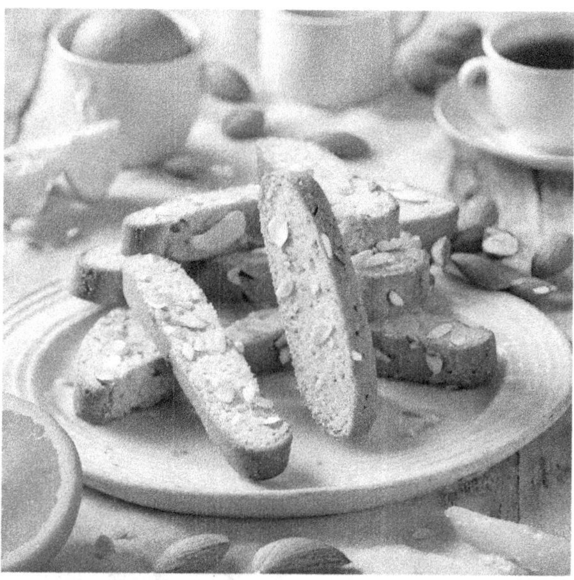

9. Blackberry and Apple Galette

Ingredients:

- 1 pie crust (homemade or store-bought)
- 2 apples, peeled, cored, and sliced
- 1 cup blackberries
- 1/4 cup sugar
- 1 tbsp cornstarch
- 1 egg, beaten for egg wash
- Sugar for sprinkling

Instructions:

1. Preheat oven to 375°F (190°C).
2. Roll out the pie crust into a circle on a parchment-lined baking sheet.
3. Toss apples, blackberries, sugar, and cornstarch together. Arrange the mixture in the center of the crust, leaving a 2-inch border.
4. Fold the edges of the crust over the filling, pleating as needed.
5. Brush the crust with egg wash and sprinkle with sugar.
6. Bake for 35-40 minutes, until the crust is golden and the filling is bubbly.
7. Serve warm.

Nutrition Info Per Serving (Serves 8):

- Calories: 210
- Fat: 9g
- Carbohydrates: 31g
- Protein: 3g
- Sodium: 110mg

Cooking Time:

- Preparation time: 20 minutes
- Cooking time: 40 minutes
- Total time: 1 hour

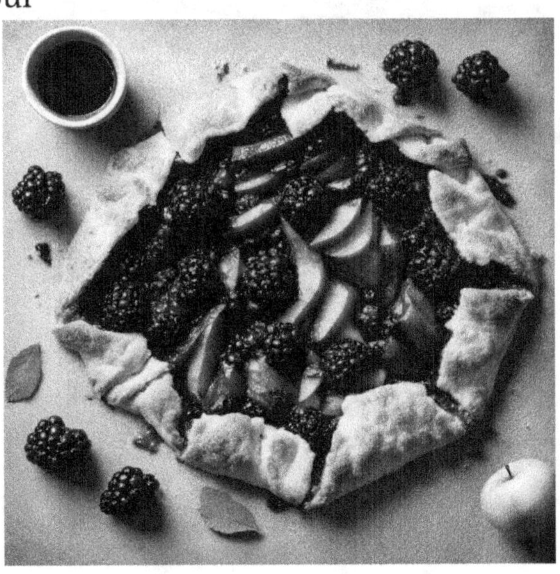

10. Kiwi and Pineapple Parfait

Ingredients:

- 2 cups Greek yogurt
- 1 cup kiwi, peeled and sliced
- 1 cup pineapple, chopped
- 2 tbsp honey
- 1/4 cup granola

Instructions:

1. In a bowl, mix Greek yogurt with honey.
2. In serving glasses, layer yogurt, kiwi slices, and pineapple chunks.
3. Repeat the layers until all ingredients are used.
4. Top each parfait with granola for crunch.
5. Serve immediately or chill until ready to serve.

Nutrition Info Per Serving (Serves 4):

- Calories: 220
- Fat: 3g
- Carbohydrates: 40g
- Protein: 10g
- Sodium: 45mg

Cooking Time:

- Preparation time: 10 minutes
- Total time: 10 minutes

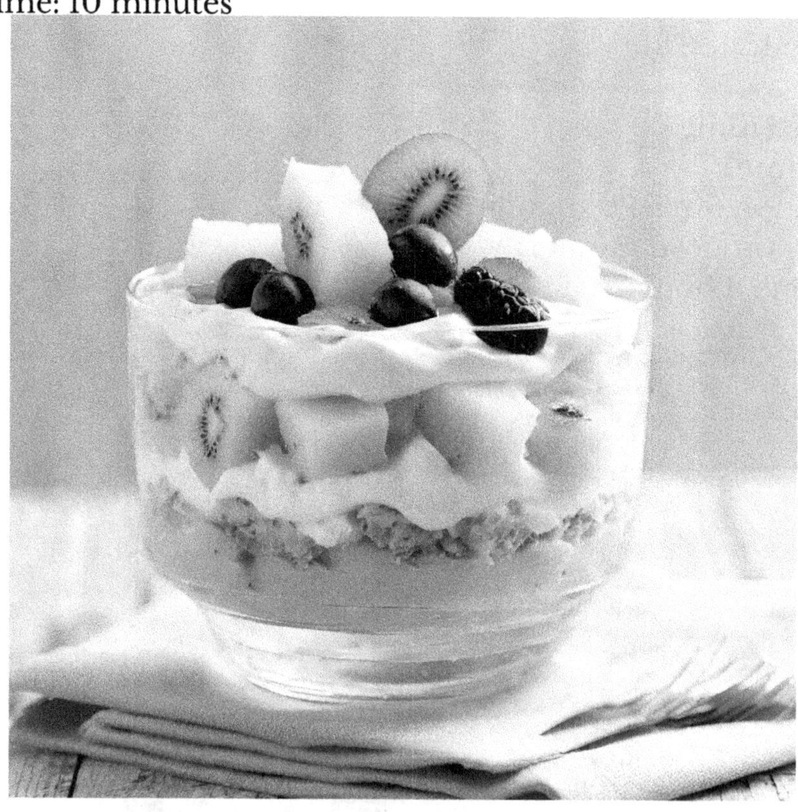

11. Vegan Chocolate Truffles

Ingredients:

- 1 cup dark chocolate chips (vegan)
- 1/2 cup coconut cream
- 1 tsp vanilla extract
- Cocoa powder, for dusting

Instructions:

1. Heat the coconut cream in a small saucepan over low heat until hot but not boiling.
2. Place chocolate chips in a bowl and pour the hot coconut cream over them. Let sit for a minute, then stir until smooth and creamy.
3. Stir in vanilla extract.
4. Refrigerate the mixture for 2-3 hours, until firm.
5. Scoop and roll into balls, then dust with cocoa powder.
6. Keep refrigerated until serving.

Nutrition Info Per Serving (Serves 12):

- Calories: 100
- Fat: 7g
- Carbohydrates: 9g
- Protein: 1g
- Sodium: 5mg

Cooking Time:

- Preparation time: 10 minutes (plus chilling)
- Total time: 3 hours 10 minutes

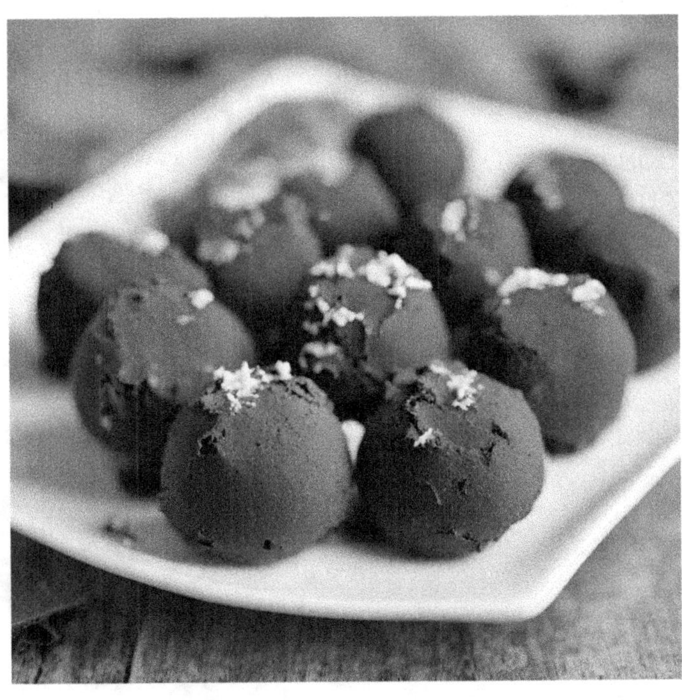

12. Strawberry Shortcake with Whipped Coconut Cream
Ingredients:

- 2 cups sliced strawberries
- 2 cups all-purpose flour
- 1/4 cup sugar, plus extra for strawberries
- 2 tsp baking powder
- 1/2 tsp salt
- 1/2 cup cold butter, cubed
- 3/4 cup milk
- 1 can coconut cream, chilled
- 1 tsp vanilla extract

Instructions:

1. Preheat oven to 425°F (220°C).
2. In a bowl, toss strawberries with a little sugar and set aside.
3. In another bowl, mix flour, 1/4 cup sugar, baking powder, and salt. Cut in butter until mixture resembles coarse crumbs. Stir in milk until dough forms.
4. Drop spoonfuls of dough onto a baking sheet. Bake for 15 minutes or until golden.
5. Meanwhile, whip chilled coconut cream with vanilla until fluffy.
6. Split shortcakes and fill with strawberries and whipped coconut cream.

Nutrition Info Per Serving (Serves 8):

- Calories: 350
- Fat: 22g
- Carbohydrates: 35g
- Protein: 4g
- Sodium: 200mg

Cooking Time:

- Preparation time: 20 minutes
- Cooking time: 15 minutes
- Total time: 35 minutes

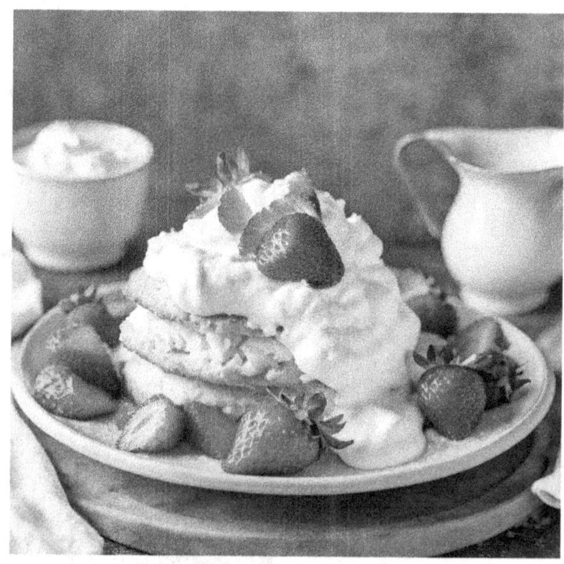

13. Blueberry Crumble with Oat Topping

Ingredients:

- 3 cups blueberries
- 1/4 cup sugar
- 1 tbsp cornstarch
- For the topping:
  - 1/2 cup rolled oats
  - 1/2 cup flour
  - 1/2 cup brown sugar
  - 1/4 cup butter, melted
  - 1/2 tsp cinnamon

Instructions:

1. Preheat oven to 375°F (190°C).
2. Mix blueberries with sugar and cornstarch, and pour into a baking dish.
3. For the topping, combine oats, flour, brown sugar, melted butter, and cinnamon until crumbly.
4. Sprinkle the oat mixture over the blueberries.
5. Bake for 30 minutes or until the topping is golden and the blueberry filling is bubbling.
6. Serve warm.

Nutrition Info Per Serving (Serves 6):

- Calories: 300
- Fat: 10g
- Carbohydrates: 50g
- Protein: 3g
- Sodium: 100mg

Cooking Time:

- Preparation time: 10 minutes
- Cooking time: 30 minutes
- Total time: 40 minutes

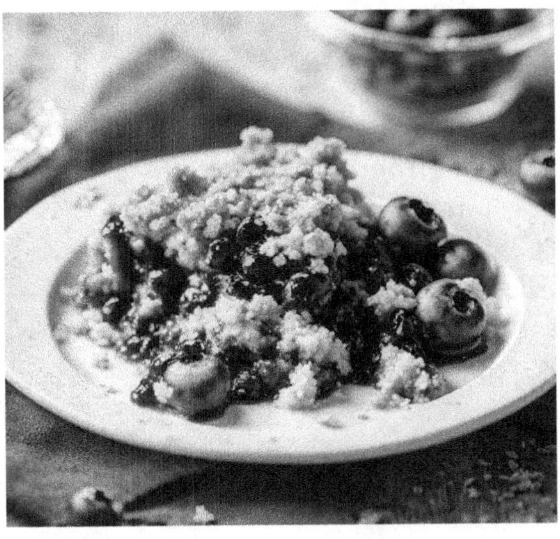

14. Raspberry and Lemon Bars

Ingredients:

- 1 1/2 cups all-purpose flour
- 1/2 cup powdered sugar, plus extra for dusting
- 3/4 cup cold butter, cubed
- 4 eggs
- 1 1/2 cups sugar
- 1/2 cup lemon juice
- 1 tbsp lemon zest
- 1/4 cup all-purpose flour
- 1/2 tsp baking powder
- 1 cup fresh raspberries

Instructions:

1. Preheat oven to 350°F (175°C). Line a 9x13 inch baking pan with parchment paper.
2. Combine 1 1/2 cups flour and 1/2 cup powdered sugar in a bowl. Cut in butter until mixture resembles coarse crumbs. Press into the bottom of the prepared pan.
3. Bake crust for 20 minutes until lightly golden.
4. In another bowl, whisk together eggs, sugar, lemon juice, and lemon zest. Mix in 1/4 cup flour and baking powder until smooth.
5. Gently fold in raspberries.
6. Pour the raspberry mixture over the baked crust.
7. Bake for an additional 25 minutes or until set.
8. Cool completely, then dust with powdered sugar before cutting into bars.

Nutrition Info Per Serving (Serves 12):

- Calories: 280
- Fat: 12g
- Carbohydrates: 40g
- Protein: 4g
- Sodium: 80mg

Cooking Time:

- Preparation time: 15 minutes
- Cooking time: 45 minutes
- Total time: 1 hour

15. Pumpkin Spice Muffins

Ingredients:

- 1 3/4 cups all-purpose flour
- 1 cup sugar
- 1/2 cup brown sugar
- 1 tsp baking soda
- 1/2 tsp salt
- 2 tsp cinnamon
- 1/4 tsp ground nutmeg
- 1/4 tsp ground cloves
- 1/4 tsp ground ginger
- 2 eggs
- 1 15 oz can pumpkin puree
- 1/2 cup vegetable oil
- 1 tsp vanilla extract

Instructions:

1. Preheat oven to 375°F (190°C). Line a muffin pan with paper liners.
2. In a large bowl, whisk together flour, sugar, brown sugar, baking soda, salt, cinnamon, nutmeg, cloves, and ginger.
3. In another bowl, mix together eggs, pumpkin puree, oil, and vanilla extract.
4. Stir the wet ingredients into the dry ingredients until just combined.
5. Scoop the batter into the prepared muffin pan, filling each cup about 3/4 full.
6. Bake for 22-25 minutes, or until a toothpick inserted into the center of a muffin comes out clean.
7. Let cool in the pan for 5 minutes, then transfer to a wire rack to cool completely.

Nutrition Info Per Serving (Serves 12):

- Calories: 290
- Fat: 11g
- Carbohydrates: 45g
- Protein: 3g
- Sodium: 200mg

Cooking Time:

- Preparation time: 15 minutes
- Cooking time: 25 minutes
- Total time: 40 minutes

6-WEEK MEAL PLAN

Week 1

Day 1
- **Breakfast:** Herbed Mushroom and Kale Frittata
- **Lunch:** Grilled Chicken with Herbs and Lemon
- **Dinner:** Beef and Broccoli Stir-Fry
- **Snack Options:** Greek Yogurt with Flaxseeds and Honey; Apple Cinnamon Bran Muffins

Day 2
- **Breakfast:** Coconut Yogurt Parfait with Mango and Pineapple
- **Lunch:** Turkey and Quinoa Stuffed Peppers
- **Dinner:** Balsamic Glazed Chicken Breast
- **Snack Options:** Almond and Orange Biscotti; Hazelnut Gelato

Day 3
- **Breakfast:** Warm Barley Cereal with Honey and Spices
- **Lunch:** Beef Bulgogi
- **Dinner:** Roasted Garlic Cauliflower
- **Snack Options:** Vegan Chocolate Truffles; Kiwi and Pineapple Parfait

Day 4
- **Breakfast:** Multi-grain Porridge with Maple Syrup and Almonds
- **Lunch:** Lamb Tagine with Apricots
- **Dinner:** Pan-Seared Trout with Walnut Gremolata
- **Snack Options:** Pomegranate and Pistachio Bark; Frozen Banana Bites Dipped in Chocolate

Day 5
- **Breakfast:** Pumpkin Oatmeal Cookies
- **Lunch:** Pork Tenderloin with Roasted Apples and Onions
- **Dinner:** Sweet Potato and Black Bean Chili
- **Snack Options:** Raspberry and Lemon Bars; Strawberry Shortcake with Whipped Coconut Cream

Day 6
- **Breakfast:** Sprouted Bean and Avocado Salad
- **Lunch:** Chicken Caesar Salad
- **Dinner:** Seared Scallops with Butternut Squash Puree
- **Snack Options:** Blackberry and Apple Galette; Blueberry Crumble with Oat Topping

Day 7
- **Breakfast:** Bulgur Wheat Pilaf with Dried Apricots and Nuts
- **Lunch:** Grilled Skirt Steak with Chimichurri Sauce
- **Dinner:** Chicken and Spinach Soup
- **Snack Options:** Pumpkin Spice Muffins; Cherry Clafoutis

Week 2

Day 1

- **Breakfast:** Steel-Cut Oats with Pumpkin Seeds and Dried Cranberries
- **Lunch:** Salmon Poke Bowl
- **Dinner:** Moroccan Lamb with Squash and Dried Plums
- **Snack Options:** Hazelnut Gelato; Raspberry and Lemon Bars

Day 2

- **Breakfast:** Whole Wheat Vegetable Pita Pocket
- **Lunch:** Roast Chicken with Garlic and Thyme
- **Dinner:** Catfish Étouffée
- **Snack Options:** Kiwi and Pineapple Parfait; Strawberry Shortcake with Whipped Coconut Cream

Day 3

- **Breakfast:** Tofu Scramble with Spinach and Sweet Peppers
- **Lunch:** Baked Sweet Potato and Poached Eggs
- **Dinner:** Vegan Chocolate Truffles
- **Snack Options:** Pumpkin Spice Muffins; Frozen Banana Bites Dipped in Chocolate

Day 4

- **Breakfast:** Savory Millet and Vegetable Bowl
- **Lunch:** Bouillabaisse with Rouille
- **Dinner:** Clam Chowder with Corn and Potatoes
- **Snack Options:** Cherry Clafoutis; Almond and Orange Biscotti

Day 5

- **Breakfast:** Mixed Berry and Flaxseed Smoothie
- **Lunch:** Beef Stew with Root Vegetables
- **Dinner:** Smoked Haddock with Pea Puree
- **Snack Options:** Blackberry and Apple Galette; Blueberry Crumble with Oat Topping

Day 6

- **Breakfast:** Pear and Ginger Compote on Ricotta Toast
- **Lunch:** Chicken Tikka Masala
- **Dinner:** Grilled Octopus with Lemon and Parsley
- **Snack Options:** Pomegranate and Pistachio Bark; Vegan Chocolate Truffles

Day 7

- **Breakfast:** Kale and White Bean Breakfast Hash
- **Lunch:** Meatloaf with Oatmeal
- **Dinner:** Fish Tacos with Cabbage Slaw
- **Snack Options:** Raspberry and Lemon Bars; Hazelnut Gelato

Week 3

Day 1
- **Breakfast**: Barley Porridge with Dates and Cardamom
- **Lunch**: Duck Breast with Cherry Sauce
- **Dinner**: Linguine with Clams and White Wine Sauce
- **Snack Options**: Kiwi and Pineapple Parfait; Cherry Clafoutis

Day 2
- **Breakfast**: Banana and Walnut Muffins (made with almond flour)
- **Lunch**: Crab-Stuffed Flounder
- **Dinner**: Turkey Meatball Soup
- **Snack Options**: Strawberry Shortcake with Whipped Coconut Cream; Frozen Banana Bites Dipped in Chocolate

Day 3
- **Breakfast**: Greek Yogurt with Flaxseeds and Honey
- **Lunch**: Vegetable Omelette with Spinach and Mushrooms
- **Dinner**: Anchovy and Tomato Flatbreads
- **Snack Options**: Blackberry and Apple Galette; Vegan Chocolate Truffles

Day 4
- **Breakfast**: Buckwheat Pancakes with Maple Syrup
- **Lunch**: Stuffed Chicken Breast with Spinach and Feta
- **Dinner**: Paella with Seafood and Saffron
- **Snack Options**: Almond and Orange Biscotti; Pumpkin Spice Muffins

Day 5
- **Breakfast**: Apple Cinnamon Bran Muffins
- **Lunch**: Baked Lemon Sole with Capers
- **Dinner**: Saffron and Cardamom Panna Cotta
- **Snack Options**: Raspberry and Lemon Bars; Pomegranate and Pistachio Bark

Day 6
- **Breakfast**: Rye Bread Avocado Toast with Tomato Slices
- **Lunch**: Spiced Turkey Burgers
- **Dinner**: Bouillabaisse with Rouille
- **Snack Options**: Blueberry Crumble with Oat Topping; Hazelnut Gelato

Day 7
- **Breakfast**: Muesli with Skim Milk and Dried Fruit
- **Lunch**: Spelt Waffles with Fresh Berries
- **Dinner**: Stuffed Bell Peppers with Quinoa and Black Beans
- **Snack Options**: Kiwi and Pineapple Parfait; Strawberry Shortcake with Whipped Coconut Cream

Week 4

Day 1
- **Breakfast**: Multi-grain Toast with Almond Butter and Banana Slices
- **Lunch**: Grilled Turkey Breast with Quinoa Salad
- **Dinner**: Lemon and Herb Roasted Salmon
- **Snack Options**: Greek Yogurt with Mixed Berries; Coconut Macaroons

Day 2
- **Breakfast**: Chia Pudding with Fresh Mango
- **Lunch**: Lentil Soup with Spinach
- **Dinner**: Garlic Lime Chicken with Asparagus
- **Snack Options**: Apple Slices with Peanut Butter; Dark Chocolate Almonds

Day 3
- **Breakfast**: Cottage Cheese with Pineapple
- **Lunch**: Veggie Wrap with Hummus
- **Dinner**: Shrimp and Asparagus Stir Fry
- **Snack Options**: Carrot Sticks with Avocado Dip; Baked Pear with Honey and Walnuts

Day 4
- **Breakfast**: Oatmeal with Chopped Pecans and Apples
- **Lunch**: Grilled Vegetable and Goat Cheese Salad
- **Dinner**: Beef Stir Fry with Broccoli and Bell Peppers
- **Snack Options**: Orange Segments; Almond Butter Energy Balls

Day 5
- **Breakfast**: Spinach and Feta Omelette
- **Lunch**: Chicken and Avocado Salad
- **Dinner**: Grilled Mackerel with Lemon Butter Sauce
- **Snack Options**: Mixed Nuts; Cottage Cheese with Sliced Peaches

Day 6
- **Breakfast**: Scrambled Eggs with Sautéed Mushrooms
- **Lunch**: Tuna Salad Stuffed Avocados
- **Dinner**: Pork Chops with Sweet Potato Mash
- **Snack Options**: Celery Sticks with Cream Cheese; Fresh Fig Halves

Day 7
- **Breakfast**: Yogurt Parfait with Granola and Kiwi
- **Lunch**: Beef and Vegetable Kabobs
- **Dinner**: Baked Cod with a Herb Crust
- **Snack Options**: Cucumber Slices with Dill Dip; Pecan Stuffed Dates

Week 5

Day 1
- **Breakfast:** Quinoa and Berry Breakfast Bowl
- **Lunch:** Spiced Grilled Chicken with Couscous Salad
- **Dinner:** Pan-Seared Sea Bass with Mediterranean Salsa
- **Snack Options:** Raspberry Coconut Balls; Peach Slices with Cottage Cheese

Day 2
- **Breakfast:** Banana Pancakes with Honey Drizzle
- **Lunch:** Moroccan Spiced Vegetable Stew
- **Dinner:** Grilled Shrimp Tacos with Cabbage Slaw
- **Snack Options:** Kiwi Fruit; Walnut and Date Bars

Day 3
- **Breakfast:** Broccoli and Cheese Frittata
- **Lunch:** Salmon and Avocado Salad
- **Dinner:** Vegan Mushroom Risotto
- **Snack Options:** Baked Apple Chips; Edamame Beans

Day 4
- **Breakfast:** Almond Milk Smoothie with Spinach and Berries
- **Lunch:** Grilled Portobello Mushroom Burger
- **Dinner:** Thai Basil Chicken
- **Snack Options:** Sliced Cucumber with Hummus; Orange Almond Biscotti

Day 5
- **Breakfast:** Sweet Potato Hash with Eggs
- **Lunch:** Spinach and Quinoa Stuffed Tomatoes
- **Dinner:** Lemon Garlic Tilapia
- **Snack Options:** Pistachio and Cranberry Bark; Yogurt with Honey and Cinnamon

Day 6
- **Breakfast:** Poached Eggs with Avocado Toast
- **Lunch:** Turkey Meatballs with Spaghetti Squash
- **Dinner:** Zucchini Noodles with Pesto and Cherry Tomatoes
- **Snack Options:** Mango Slices; Spiced Roasted Chickpeas

Day 7
- **Breakfast:** Protein Shake with Mixed Berries
- **Lunch:** Roasted Beet and Feta Salad
- **Dinner:** Chicken Stuffed Peppers
- **Snack Options:** Apple and Almond Butter Slices; Olives and Cheese

Week 6

Day 1
- **Breakfast**: Granola with Skim Milk and Blueberries
- **Lunch**: Egg Salad on Whole Grain Bread
- **Dinner**: Stuffed Aubergines with Lamb and Pine Nuts
- **Snack Options**: Pear with Almond Paste; Flaxseed and Oat Crackers

Day 2
- **Breakfast**: Green Smoothie with Kale, Banana, and Almond Milk
- **Lunch**: Chicken and Mango Chutney Sandwich
- **Dinner**: Grilled Halibut with a Pineapple Salsa
- **Snack Options**: Raw Carrots with Tahini; Dried Apricots and Walnuts

Day 3
- **Breakfast**: French Toast with Strawberries
- **Lunch**: Avocado and Sprout Salad
- **Dinner**: Spaghetti with Clam Sauce
- **Snack Options**: Greek Yogurt with Pomegranate; Baked Sweet Potato Fries

Day 4
- **Breakfast**: Muesli with Almond Milk
- **Lunch**: Caesar Salad with Grilled Chicken
- **Dinner**: Moroccan Tagine with Fish
- **Snack Options**: Baked Banana with Cinnamon; Sunflower Seeds

Day 5
- **Breakfast**: Buckwheat Pancakes with Maple Syrup
- **Lunch**: Vegetable Lasagna
- **Dinner**: Grilled Swordfish with Herb Butter
- **Snack Options**: Chilled Melon Soup; Cashew Nut Brittle

Day 6
- **Breakfast**: Egg White Omelet with Spinach and Tomatoes
- **Lunch**: Quinoa Tabbouleh
- **Dinner**: Lamb Chops with Mint Pesto
- **Snack Options**: Roasted Almonds; Baked Pear with Cinnamon

Day 7
- **Breakfast**: Oatmeal with Fresh Fruit and Nuts
- **Lunch**: Grilled Vegetable Platter with Tzatziki
- **Dinner**: Duck Breast with Orange Sauce
- **Snack Options**: Carrot and Celery Sticks with Blue Cheese Dip; Fresh Figs with Ricotta

WEEKLY MEAL PLANNER 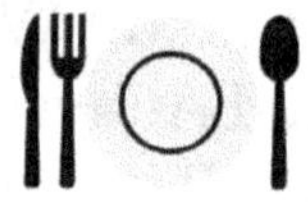

	BREAKFAST	LUNCH	DINNER	SNACKS
MONDAY				
TUESDAY				
WEDNESDAY				
THURSDAY				
FRIDAY				
SATURDAY				
SUNDAY				

What specific goals do you hope to achieve by following this hyperthyroidism diet? (e.g., symptom relief, weight management)

WEEKLY MEAL PLANNER 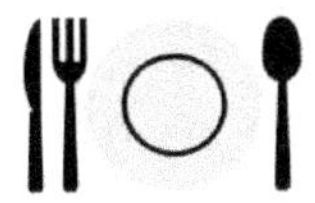

	BREAKFAST	LUNCH	DINNER	SNACKS
MONDAY				
TUESDAY				
WEDNESDAY				
THURSDAY				
FRIDAY				
SATURDAY				
SUNDAY				

ave you tried any diets or foods in the past that seemed to improve or worsen your symptoms? What were they?

WEEKLY MEAL PLANNER 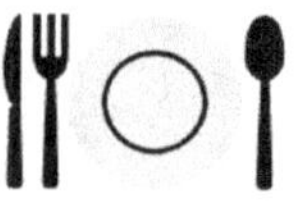

	BREAKFAST	LUNCH	DINNER	SNACKS
MONDAY				
TUESDAY				
WEDNESDAY				
THURSDAY				
FRIDAY				
SATURDAY				
SUNDAY				

What are your expectations from the hyperthyroidism diet? What changes do you hope to see in your symptoms?

WEEKLY MEAL PLANNER 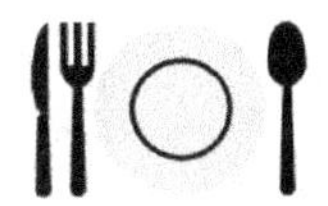

	BREAKFAST	LUNCH	DINNER	SNACKS
MONDAY				
TUESDAY				
WEDNESDAY				
THURSDAY				
FRIDAY				
SATURDAY				
SUNDAY				

Do you feel equipped to plan your meals according to the hyperthyroidism diet guidelines? What challenges do you anticipate?

WEEKLY MEAL PLANNER 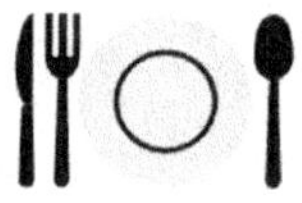

	BREAKFAST	LUNCH	DINNER	SNACKS
MONDAY				
TUESDAY				
WEDNESDAY				
THURSDAY				
FRIDAY				
SATURDAY				
SUNDAY				

Besides dietary changes, what other lifestyle modifications are you considering to manage your hyperthyroidism?

WEEKLY MEAL PLANNER

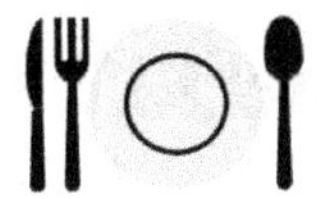

	BREAKFAST	LUNCH	DINNER	SNACKS
MONDAY				
TUESDAY				
WEDNESDAY				
THURSDAY				
FRIDAY				
SATURDAY				
SUNDAY				

How comfortable are you with identifying foods that are considered beneficial or detrimental to thyroid health?

WEEKLY MEAL PLANNER

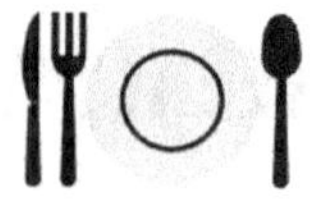

	BREAKFAST	LUNCH	DINNER	SNACKS
MONDAY				
TUESDAY				
WEDNESDAY				
THURSDAY				
FRIDAY				
SATURDAY				
SUNDAY				

How willing and able are you to adapt your current favorite recipes to fit the hyperthyroidism diet?

WEEKLY MEAL PLANNER 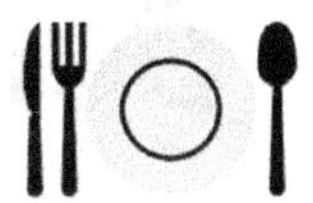

	BREAKFAST	LUNCH	DINNER	SNACKS
MONDAY				
TUESDAY				
WEDNESDAY				
THURSDAY				
FRIDAY				
SATURDAY				
SUNDAY				

If your initial dietary adjustments don't yield the expected benefits, how do you plan to further modify your approach?

Please Scan this QR Code to Get Your Bonus Content